THE ULTIMATE GIFT

Also by Roy Calne

The Gift of Life
Too Many People
Art, Surgery and Transplantation

THE ULTIMATE GIFT

The Story of Britain's Premier Transplant Surgeon

Roy Calne

HEADLINE

First published in 1998
by HEADLINE BOOK PUBLISHING

10 9 8 7 6 5 4 3 2 1

British Library Cataloguing in Publication Data

Calne, Roy Yorke, 1930-
The ultimate gift: the story of Britain's
premier transplant surgeon
1.Calne, Roy Yorke, 1930-
2.Surgeons - Great Britain - Biography
I.Title
617.9'5'092

ISBN 0 7472 2043 3

Typeset by
Letterpart Limited, Reigate, Surrey

Printed and bound in Great Britain by
Mackays of Chatham PLC, Chatham, Kent

HEADLINE BOOK PUBLISHING
A division of Hodder Headline PLC
338 Euston Road
London NW1 3BH

To the transplant patients and their donors

Contents

Acknowledgements	ix
Introduction	xi
Chapter One: Because It Can't Be Done	1
Chapter Two: Ukuleles, Gurkhas and a Painted Virgin	11
Chapter Three: The Shoulders of Giants	21
Chapter Four: Into the Unknown	37
Chapter Five: New Horizons	45
Chapter Six: Other People's Organs	55
Chapter Seven: The Cambridge Connection	73
Chapter Eight: Crossing the Rubicon	93
Chapter Nine: The Search for New Drugs	115
Chapter Ten: The Media Circus	123
Chapter Eleven: Home and Abroad	135
Chapter Twelve: The Art of Surgery	147
Chapter Thirteen: Successes and Shortcomings	157
Chapter Fourteen: Crystal Ball Gazing	177
Appendix I: The Main Transplant Organs	191
Appendix II: Glossary	199
Appendix III: Key Dates in the History of Transplantation	201
Index	203

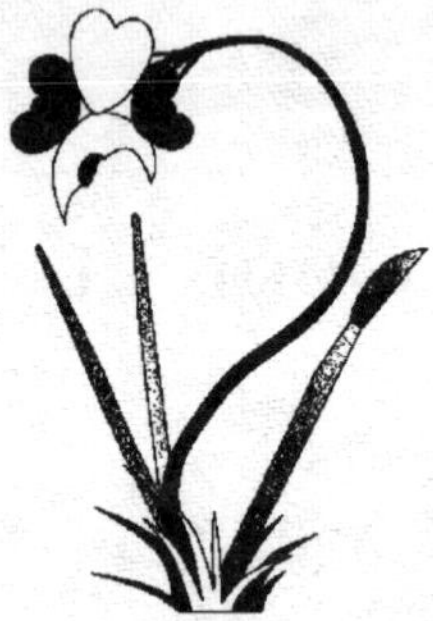

The 'transplant' – an orchid with petals of kidneys, heart and liver and leaves of forceps and a scalpel.

Acknowledgements

I would like to acknowledge the unending work and advice I have received from Cathy Riethoff, who has devoted a great deal of her energy and interest to this book. Thanks to my wife, family and colleagues for contributing to the recollections and anecdotes. I am especially grateful to my wife for repeatedly reading the manuscript and for providing constructive criticism. My thanks to Medical Photography at Addenbrooke's for their help with the illustrations; and to Celia Kent, Kelly Davis and Barbara Kiser and their colleagues at Headline for their work on the text and to Liz Cadman for her proof reading skills. My thanks also to Alan Brooke for giving me the initial idea of writing this book.

Introduction

This is both a personal story and an account of the evolution of a new form of life-saving medical treatment. Organ transplantation was summarily dismissed as impossible when I was a student, but has now become a routine and usually successful enterprise.

The journey has not been easy. We have often taken wrong turnings and, even when we thought we were following the correct path, new hazards have suddenly appeared. Success has bred unexpected and intractable moral dilemmas, and success is still only partial.

Centre stage are the patients facing death due to failure of a vital organ, welcoming new and unproven treatment with great courage but also with no positive alternative. A functioning organ must come from a living volunteer donor or a recently dead person. Generous sacrifice or sudden tragedy are therefore the backdrops to each transplant operation. Questions never before asked in medicine intrude constantly in the transplant dialogue. How can death be diagnosed confidently so that the organs can be removed while they are still usable? Who can and should give permission for organ donation? How can the dignity of the dying patient and the grieving relatives be preserved when organ removal is contemplated?

Who can volunteer to give an organ and to whom? Should a child be allowed to give a kidney to her identical twin, or a husband to his wife? The shortage of donor organs and the success of transplantation have vastly increased the waiting lists. Many doctors cry out for more to be done but to receive an organ graft is a privilege and not a right. Should a self-inflicted disease, such as alcoholism, exclude a patient from the liver transplant waiting list? How should society judge the sale of organs, or the removal of organs from executed prisoners? How can we prevent the stealing of organs, or even murder for organs? Two hundred years ago people were murdered to provide bodies for dissection.

Ethics are defined by the way society regards the practice in question. In medieval times Western society accepted torture and execution as an ethical way of dealing with religious heretics, and the world is still not entirely free of this prejudice. Would organ transplantation from animals to man be considered ethical if it could save human lives? Is it morally right for rich Western nations to spend vast sums on high-tech medicine and surgery for a few patients, while millions live in poverty without any medical care at all?

I shall try to examine all these matters from a personal viewpoint, as one who has been involved in organ transplantation from its beginnings, though I must admit that clear-cut answers are seldom forthcoming.

The biology of organ grafting remains a fascinating subject. How does the body react when another's tissues are abruptly joined to its own? How can we make this coming together friendly and beneficial to the sick patient? Can the body's tendency to reject organ grafts be controlled by less harmful means than those we use at present?

In this book I will explain what has happened so far: what we know and, more important, what we don't yet know. I will recount the individual histories of research pioneers and their discoveries; and I will record tales of courage and perseverance in the face of adversity, of patients who have struggled in vain and others who have triumphed. All have conquered fear and pain, confronting the hazards of a procedure that is no longer considered impossible.

Roy Calne

Chapter One

Because It Can't Be Done

He was nearly the same colour as his sheets, a greyish white; his legs were swollen, his tongue dry and furred, and his breath had a stale, putrefying odour. It was 1950, I was a medical student at Guy's Hospital, and this boy, one of my patients, was dying of kidney failure after developing the dreaded Bright's disease. It was this – the sight of Jonathan and other young people dying from the simple lack of a functioning organ – that triggered my interest in transplantation.

A large group of us, ten students, two house physicians and junior and senior registrars, had followed the consultant from bed to bed on our round through the long, spotless 'Nightingale' wards. We had surrounded Jonathan's bed, and I, facing the consultant, presented the history and clinical examination. The consultant, after confirming the diagnosis of Bright's disease and ushering us away from the bed, then told the ward sister that we should make the boy as comfortable as possible because he would die in the next two weeks. We had studied anatomy and dissected the whole body, and I knew that the kidneys were vital organs, with a large blood flow made necessary by their function as filters.

Each kidney had one large artery and an even larger vein. The urine drained through a sizeable tube, the ureter. The connections were so simple, so why not graft a kidney into the patient?

Jonathan was my patient, and I was permitted to ask a question:

'Since the only cause of his illness is kidney failure, can he have a kidney graft?'

There was an ominous silence. The consultant looked a little angry and replied, 'No.'

Oblivious to the obvious signs that I was entering a 'no-go' area, I asked very politely, 'Why not?'

A terse 'Because it can't be done' was the end of the matter.

I was about to put my head further into the noose and ask why, but one of my friends tugged my arm and whispered, 'If you want a house job at Guy's, shut up!'

At tea in the students' cafeteria afterwards we argued about this preposterous idea. Surely a surgeon could join the artery, vein and ureter of a donor kidney to the artery, vein and ureter of the patient – but what would happen then? Our lectures and textbooks said nothing about such revolutionary proposals. I watched Jonathan's terrible decline, assuaged partly by the merciful Brompton Mixture (morphia, cocaine and brandy), until he lapsed into a coma and died, a failure of our care. I was unaware that even then, in 1950, the surgical techniques of kidney transplantation were being developed in Boston in the United States, and that the biology of transplantation was being unravelled under the critical and curious eye of that master of transplantation immunology, Peter Medawar, in London. Soon after, the need to study for finals and obtain house jobs obliterated my latent interest in organ grafting.

Rebellious Roots

Nine years later I was to embark on a journey of research and experimentation that would ultimately lead to my work on organ transplantation. It was a risk, since in 1959 there was no clinical organ grafting in humans as we now know it, but my nature has always been rebellious.

According to my mother, I was difficult as a child, and did not respond easily to the normal persuasive tactics of parents, even when they included force. Thus, when I was five, after I had perpetrated a number of consistently anti-social acts, my father – normally a mild man, but sometimes angry when provoked – locked me in the cellar of our house in Richmond, Surrey. He was surprised to see me appearing shortly afterwards with minor cuts, and found the cellar window shattered.

Hand in hand with this rebelliousness went a fascination with nature and mechanical things. I wanted to know all about animals, plants and engines. My father must have inspired some of this interest, as he was very skilful with his hands and also very inventive. As a youth he had been an apprentice car engineer at the Rover Car Company in Coventry, where he learned the 'anatomy' and 'surgery' of the internal combustion engine. He was ambitious and after his apprenticeship he sailed to America to learn the advanced manufacturing and business methods of Detroit. He eventually moved to Richmond. My mother, by contrast, had a quiet temperament. She was passionately interested in education, and so had been bitterly disappointed when, after matriculating, she found that her parents could not afford to send her to university. It was her ambition that her children *would* get this chance, and she was a severe tutor to my younger brother and myself.

At the age of eight, I was due to go to a London preparatory school, Colet Court. But with the outbreak of the Second World War, the school was evacuated to a country estate near Marlow, in the Thames Valley, and we were accommodated in a palatial house belonging to the biscuit millionaire Garfield Weston. The grounds had streams and trees and bordered on the River Thames – a boon both for my interest in nature and my mischievous tendencies, as at this time two friends and I managed to borrow a punt and actually manoeuvre it out on the river. We were swept over the weir in Marlow, beside the Compleat Angler Hotel, stranded miles from the school, and finally rescued by the occupants of a powerful motorboat. We scrambled into the classroom just in time for evening school. I have always had an affection for the Compleat Angler Hotel since then, as a symbol of our rescue.

The war kept us all on the move, and soon, when my father found a job assembling imported American jeeps in North Wales, we went to live in a little terraced house in Old Colwyn. Here we spent the rest of the war years. I attended three different schools, ending up at Dulwich College prep school, which had been evacuated to Betws-y-Coed, an idyllic spot in the mountains, near the River Conway.

My scholastic achievements at school were modest, except in biology where I did rather better. I was fascinated by the anatomy and physiology of animals and plants, and particularly enjoyed drawing zoology and botany specimens. The main educational benefit of the school, however, was its clear demonstration to us, at an early age, that the world was an unfair place, punishments were arbitrary, and effort seldom rewarded. Acceptance of this pattern of human behaviour was a useful lesson to take away from school: it made us realists.

At the age of twelve I was told by the headmaster at Dulwich College to sit scholarship papers for a variety of public schools, since my parents could not afford to pay for me. After writing a number of examination papers I was delighted and surprised to be awarded a minor scholarship to Lancing College on the Sussex Downs, a school I had never heard of. My parents were pleased and my father took me on a long walk by the Conway to discuss my future.

He knew that I was fascinated by biology, but also by things mechanical, and I think he would have liked me to follow him into the motor business. But I explained to him that, interesting as the internal combustion engine was, I thought the human engine was probably the more fascinating phenomenon. I told my father that I would like to continue with my scientific studies and eventually specialise in medicine, and I clearly remember expressing a desire to be a surgeon, although I knew nothing of surgery except that it involved solving problems by the use of one's hands. He accepted this, and both he and my mother gave me strong and continuing encouragement.

In the meantime Lancing was evacuated to Shropshire, near the town of Ludlow, and not until the war's end in 1945 did the college – along with me and the rest of the boarders – move back to its magnificent location on the Sussex Downs. The school building there is an extremely beautiful example of the late Victorian neo-Gothic revival. And, overall, I enjoyed my few years there, although I do have memories of freezing winters and an empty stomach.

My interest in nature and the life sciences grew, as our housemaster was an amateur biologist and microscopist who encouraged us to keep animals. I was particularly fascinated by birds, and kept a flock of forty pigeons, which I had reared from squealing chicks collected from the attic of the college chapel, above the beautiful vaulted domes. Pigeons used the attic's wooden planks as roosting spots; most were carrier pigeons who, after crossing the Channel, became tired or buffeted by winds. For them, the chapel was a peaceful escape from the hard life of competitive racing. I also kept jackdaws, rooks and magpies. The only birds that I was unable to tame were two beautiful barn owls. When they were old enough, I set them free, and I think they were glad to see the back of me; the feeling was mutual.

In at the Deep End

At sixteen, exhilarated after coping with the school certificate, I was granted an interview for entrance to Guy's Hospital Medical School as a student. I was immensely pleased – not least because I'd had enough of school. I think my tutors at Lancing were surprised when I was accepted. The headmaster at first felt it would be inadvisable for me to go to medical school at such a young age. However, on second thoughts he agreed, his *volte-face* almost certainly influenced by the thought of otherwise having to put up with me for another year at Lancing.

At the interview at Guy's I was asked the usual question: why did I want to be a doctor and go to Guy's? I gave the expected answers, but omitted to mention that London Bridge train station, which is adjacent to Guy's, was on the direct route to Epsom Downs station, close to our family house. The interviewing panel seemed to be very impressed with the fact that I was in the middle of reading *Pride and Prejudice.*

So I was in; but I had little idea at that point what I was in for. Life as a medical student in London in 1947 was not very pleasant. I commuted from home, except when I was on duty, in the clinical years and that train journey gave me time to do at least two hours' work every day. I was able to immerse myself in my books and ignore the bustle of the crowds.

Unlike Oxford and Cambridge, where tutors paid a great deal of attention to the needs, worries and general progress of undergraduates, Guy's was a sink-or-swim sort of place. You attended the lectures and practical classes and took the exams. If you passed you moved to clinical; if you failed you had one more chance; and if you failed again you were out. Nobody was the least bit interested in your personal worries, girlfriends, troubles with work or home environment.

After completing anatomy, physiology and pharmacology and passing the exams, we moved into the wards as clinical students. Now life became moving and exciting: there were real people, distressed and ill, for whom we students had direct responsibility. We took their histories, examined them and became their own personal, if ignorant, 'doctors'. We were allowed to do minor surgical procedures and even emergency surgery, which was particularly challenging when we were the first to deal with victims of severe accidents.

I remember once when Paul Large, our senior registrar, the 'Crown Prince' of the surgical hierarchy, was leading the senior dressers (who were responsible for changing dressings) and junior ward clerks (who wrote up patients' histories and symptoms) across the park at Guy's, he suddenly stopped. Solemnly pointing to the medical block, Hunts House, he turned to us and said, 'There you see before you an edifice dedicated to bullshit.' He went on:

> Unlike surgeons, physicians just talk, but we have to act and treat the patients. If we make an error, we and everybody know about it and we have to decide to operate or not to operate and what operations to do. We often have little information and are under the stress of time with a rapidly

> deteriorating patient. The physicians prescribe a drug, and if that doesn't work, another drug, so if the patient gets better that is due to their brilliance, whereas if the patient gets worse it is the will of God.

So saying, he led us off to an acute surgical emergency. It was a salutary speech.

When I became a senior surgical student, I elected to join the prestigious cardiac surgical firm of Mr Russell Brock. He was a figure of international repute, and an outstanding surgical anatomist and pathologist with a clinical acumen that was legendary. Brock was of average height, with dark hair and a serious, tight-lipped expression. He had a sense of humour which was difficult to find but it did come out at certain moments. However, he was terrifying to work with in the operating theatre.

At that time Brock had just started operating on valves, particularly the mitral valve, the main one on the left side of the heart. He was engaging in procedures that had never been done before. Many of the patients died: I once assisted with a valve operation on a young girl who died shortly after the operation because the valve could not be reached. At the next ward round, he had a little gleaming knife, attached to a ring that fitted on his little finger, which he had designed and made since the operation a few days before. He held up this knife for us to see, pointed to the empty bed and said, 'If I had had this miniature knife last week the child in this bed would still be alive.'

He was very critical of himself, always striving for improvement. He would put his finger in the chamber of a patient's heart and feel the valve to determine whether or not it was diseased and what needed to be done. Then, standing in the operating theatre with his finger inside the left atrium of the heart, he would turn around to the assembled company and say that, while the cardiologists had insisted there was no mitral regurgitation (or back flow of blood when the main ventricle contracted), 'I can, however, feel a powerful jet of blood impinging onto my finger. It's a pity they are not here to feel it themselves.'

I hero-worshipped Brock, who displayed an obsessive attention to detail in the care of his patients. The rest of his team were no less formidable. Sister Faulwasser, his ward sister, who lived in a little room on the ward, was a member of the Plymouth Brethren. She was gaunt, thin and severe but she willed patients to live, and had a sixth sense of when things were beginning to go wrong. She would say to a nurse, 'Go to Mr Jones, he is going to vomit' before he vomited; or 'You'd better get the registrar, Mr Smith is about to die.' She would say, 'Go and see Mr Johnson, I think he is bleeding internally,' and she would be right. She was like all the monitors in an intensive care ward put together, without the cables. This type of nurse is not to be found today. She was a strict disciplinarian – respected and feared by patients, nurses and doctors.

The senior registrar, Ben Milstein, was also a hard taskmaster who expected his students to be perceptive and knowledgeable. On one occasion, my response to a question halted his flow of words. He then enquired whether I could drive a tractor, 'because there may be a career for you in farming that would be suitable, since you are obviously ill equipped to become a doctor'.

Shifting Dullness and Sudden Emergencies

The most prestigious house jobs were at Guy's Hospital but I had serious doubts that I would get one. Nevertheless, after I finally qualified as a doctor (gaining a distinction in medicine but not in surgery, despite my preference), I was fortunate enough to get a job as a house physician at Guy's. The mess life there was enjoyable, but the ward rounds were dull and interminable and known to the students as 'shifting dullness' (the name given to the percussion sound when an abdomen containing fluid is moved from side to side). I was therefore very excited to move to a general surgical job under Mr Eckhoff, a tall, distinguished-looking South African who had been a formidable rugby player.

As his students, we had once invited him to a firm dinner at one of the local pubs and he had driven up in his Rolls and parked outside. He was good company and we decided it would be fun to make him drunk. He downed whisky for whisky with us, but, one after another, we students gave up the contest in waves of nausea and oblivion. Having survived trial by alcohol, Mr Eckhoff stood up, smiled, thanked everybody for a delightful evening, got into his Rolls and drove off. He was a careful and gentle surgeon and I had a deep respect for him, not only for his amusing and comradely social presence, but for his devoted and skilful care of his patients.

During this general surgical post, I was woken one night by the porter (we didn't have phones in our rooms), and told that I had to go and give an anaesthetic. According to the rules of the hospital, if there was no anaesthetist available, the house surgeon on duty had to give anaesthetics to patients in labour anywhere in the area around the hospital. So I soon found myself, together with the midwife on duty (a stern, middle-aged lady, dressed in uniform with a black cape), bicycling off to a tenement building not far from Guy's. The anaesthetist's bag consisted of a simple mask which looked like a sieve, gauze, a bottle of chloroform and a bottle of ether. I had been taught to use ether, and warned that chloroform was extremely dangerous and could kill patients. But to my horror, when we arrived in the room where the woman with an obstructed labour lay, not only were things going badly, but the sole source of heat was an open fire. I knew that ether was inflammable, but had to make a decision quickly because the obstetric registrar was coming to apply forceps.

I took out the mask, held it over her face, and sprinkled chloroform on the gauze. She immediately went into deep unconsciousness. I thought I had killed her, so I took the mask off. She very quickly woke up and vomited fish and chips all over me and the bed. I returned to the task of anaesthetising her while the baby was extracted safely. There was a crying bundle and the smell of vomit and worse. I was glad that I had decided to do surgery and not obstetrics.

My next job was as house surgeon to Mr Brock – a difficult post, as I was often up all night with desperately ill patients. The mortality rate was high and it was a dreadful feeling when a patient died and I had to phone Brock up and tell him the news. He was always sympathetic and thanked me for the effort I had made, even if it had been in vain.

On one occasion, a ten-year-old girl was admitted to the ward. She was a deep purple blue with club-shaped fingers; a loud noise like a diesel engine could be heard when listening to her heart. She had an abnormal connection between the two main arteries supplying the body – a 'patent ductus'. This can usually be corrected by a simple operation to tie off the bypass artery. However, this girl had presented late and she was operated on when the flow of blood had reversed. This was why she was blue – patients with this condition are generally a normal colour. Sadly, when the abnormal duct was tied off she did not make a complete recovery as had been expected. Instead she got progressively weaker until her heart failed. This was a serious warning to us to operate on these patients as early as possible.

In the operating theatre Brock was difficult to assist and he seemed to generate a high level of tension. When I was a medical student, he once handed me a piece of bent tubing. It was customary to call medical students 'doctor' in derision, and Brock said, 'This, doctor, is a sucker. When you see blood there, you suck.' I was terrified and held the sucker in my shaking hand. A little blood appeared and I thrust the sucker into the patient's chest to aspirate the blood. Brock swung round at me and shouted, 'Don't threaten me with that instrument!' I withdrew it, shaking even more. Some more blood appeared, until eventually there was quite a puddle. I hesitated – then Brock turned on me again, yelling, 'Don't you see there's blood there? Suck! What do you think you are, an ornament?' Yet he taught me the important lesson that one should always listen carefully to what the patient has to say, and always to try to correlate their physical signs and symptoms with the relevant anatomical and physiological abnormalities. He was a kindly, generous and hospitable man outside the operating theatre and in later years we became friends.

Chapter Two

Ukuleles, Gurkhas and a Painted Virgin

During my first house jobs, I had, in a sense, been living on borrowed time. My National Service had been deferred because of medical studies, but now I had to face it – two years as a medical officer in the Royal Army Medical Corps (RAMC).

We went to Aldershot for the preliminary training, square bashing and indoctrination into the mysterious ways of the military. Most of my group wished to stay in the UK, as this was thought to be the best way of obtaining good jobs after National Service. I was the only cadet who wished to go abroad. Usually the army goes out of its way to ensure that you don't get your choice of postings, but in my case the commanding officer was so pleased that one of the cadets wished to leave the UK that he confirmed my posting to Singapore.

When departure was imminent, we slept in a converted barrack area deep beneath London, in Goodge Street Underground station. After several false alarms, in January of 1953 we were driven in army trucks to Northolt Airport, where our transport was an exceedingly noisy and uncomfortable Lancaster Bomber. The first stop was Rome, where I managed to purchase a flagon of Chianti. This somewhat softened the journey to the next stop, Bahrain, and then it was on to Karachi, where we spent the first night in an ancient hotel with a ceiling fan pulled by a servant. The curry gave us all severe abdominal pain and diarrhoea, a state of affairs that did not improve at Delhi, the terminus of the next leg of our journey.

Tea with Curry Powder

We finally arrived at Singapore, where I was posted as a surgeon to the British military hospital. After a few months there, I was sent to Hong Kong without any warning, and eventually landed what was considered a plum posting – doctor to a Gurkha regiment in the New Territories, on the border with China. The Scottish medical officer who was leaving advised me to buy a ukulele, as he felt that learning a musical instrument would help me while away hours of boredom. I took his advice and became a modest performer on the instrument, managing to produce a fairly large repertoire of songs, mostly of a dubious nature.

This was a vital and enjoyable time for me. Anyone who has worked with the Gurkhas has a deep admiration and love for them. Such continuous cheerfulness and fierce loyalty are rarely encountered. They were passionate, too – first about women, secondly about drinking, thirdly about gambling and fourthly about fighting. Their love of women caused some complications in my surgery: my Indian nurse confessed to me, 'Doctor Sahib, so much beauty is a terrible trial and a burden to bear, in this regiment.' (She was curvaceous and beautiful but she would still have had a hard time even if she had been ugly!)

My predecessor told me before he went that all the official medical equipment was in a locked and sealed trunk which I was on no account ever to touch, let alone use. All our day-to-day equipment had been a gift from the quartermaster, following the last hurricane. (Hurricanes were like manna from heaven to him because he could write down that everything had been destroyed, including the things that had been lost or purloined.)

I was assigned a batman, called an orderly, who looked after my personal needs: he stood behind me at mealtimes, ran my bath and looked after my uniform and equipment. Every morning he would bring me a pint mug of tea with curry powder in it – revolting to taste the first time, but after a few weeks a lack of curry powder made tea taste like water. In the mess, breakfast always consisted of mulligatawny soup, to which we could add, if we wished, further chillies and sherry. The Gurkha officers would invite their British colleagues to drinks in their mess, offering rough and very powerful Indian rum accompanied by hot green chillies instead of biscuits.

Idyllic as this time was, certain frustrations plagued me. There was, for instance, a young Gurkha recruit who came to sick parade coughing blood and short of breath, with a high temperature. A chest x-ray confirmed that he had tuberculosis, an affliction to which the Gurkhas were especially prone when they came down from the mountains of their homeland to sea level. I prescribed streptomycin for him, but was then told, in a directive from the RAMC in Hong Kong, that streptomycin could only be prescribed for British soldiers. I complained bitterly, and said that my MP might find this an interesting subject to discuss in the House of Commons. The next day, the streptomycin was sent – but my popularity with the upper echelons of the hierarchy plummeted.

Other directives were equally arbitrary and strange. For example, I had a mule at my disposal for night-time exercises, but I wasn't allowed to ride on it. It carried the forbidden, locked trunk containing the medical equipment. The mule knew exactly where to put its feet, even on a pitch black night with no stars or moon. It never faltered or fell, which was more than could be said of us soldiers, particularly myself, who had not had the benefit of the rigorous infantry discipline which the rest had experienced.

After a few months settling in with the Gurkhas, I was suddenly issued with a posting to Japan, again out of the blue. I had mixed feelings about going to Japan, not just because of the war, but also because I was so content with the Gurkhas. The night before my departure, my friends at 33rd General Hospital threw a party for me, which was noisy, enjoyable and somewhat rebellious. Afterwards I drove back to the New Territories in my ancient Sunbeam Alpine. On the outskirts of the city of Kowloon, I was stopped by a policeman, who wasn't interested in how much I had had to drink, but wondered if I could give him a lift to his village which was next to our camp. I was happy to do so and the two of us enjoyed the fresh air of the Hong Kong night in my open car.

The next day I bade farewell to my friends in the 2nd Goorkhas and was driven by jeep to a troop ship in Hong Kong harbour, bound for Japan. Shortly before the ship was due to sail, there was a loud commotion in the corridor. Two military policemen burst into my stateroom, followed by a colonel who informed me that I was under arrest. The charge was quite clear: I was being arrested for painting a statue of the Virgin Mary outside 33rd General Hospital with gentian violet dye.

Apparently a fairly extensive paint job had been done and nobody knew how to remove the offending pigment. I was marched before the senior Colonel of the RAMC who explained the details of the charge. My simple statement that I knew nothing about the painting and that I wasn't even aware that the statue existed was received with disbelief by the Colonel. However, I suddenly remembered the policeman to whom I had given a lift on the outskirts of Kowloon and the fact that the painting had taken place several hours after my departure. The Colonel permitted the Military Police to make a search for the policeman. He was easily found, since I knew where he lived, and he confirmed the times that I had picked him up and dropped him off, thus establishing my innocence.

By this time my ship was well on its way to Japan, and I had to be re-posted back to my Gurkha regiment, much to my joy. Two weeks later Patsy, my future wife, arrived in Hong Kong, so that bizarre false accusation was a marvellous stroke of fate. And the true culprit? Much later, a pathology technician informed me – at top decibel from the porthole of a retreating troop ship – that his was the offending hand.

An Exotic Honeymoon

Patsy had been a nurse at Guy's and when I was house surgeon she had come under my care with appendicitis, and I had assisted at the removal of her appendix. I had a chance to inspect her from within, and so knew that everything was all right. She was by far the most beautiful nurse at the hospital and we had been friends for some time, although we were not actually engaged. Patsy had joined the army at the same time as me, and had had to sign on for three years in order to get a posting to the East.

When she arrived on the troop plane, she was like a princess descending from the sky, and after a whirlwind courtship we decided to get married. Our wedding day was planned for the eve of the departure of our regiment for Malaya – another sudden army move in a short spell of time. We were married from the regiment, I in full military regalia, and our honeymoon was spent on the *SS Tchwangi*, a beautiful Dutch steamboat which took us through the South China Seas to Singapore.

The regiment was posted to Kuala Pilah, a village deep in the jungle in the midst of bandit country: the Gurkhas were very good at jungle fighting and welcomed the opportunity to engage in active service. It was a vicious campaign, with no quarter given by either side. Both the Gurkhas and the Chinese terrorists were extremely brave and determined – 'shoot to kill' was the motto on both sides. Patsy and another officer's wife had a small flat in the town of Seremban, and I would motor from there in my old Sunbeam at a furious speed to Kuala Pilah. Patsy and her friend became very worried: at night they frequently heard strange noises below their house, which had a large cellar, and feared that it could be communist activity. When the matter was investigated by the local police, however, it appeared that the owner of the house used the basement as a highly successful brothel. Relative quiet was established thereafter.

Such excitements were only part of the story. More mundane problems also dogged us. As I was doing National Service, I was not entitled to a marriage allowance, yet the dearth of hospital jobs up-country in Malaya made it extremely difficult for Patsy to find work and we were very short of money. I would stuff my pockets in the mess with rolls and bits and pieces of food to bring back to her. This situation was only resolved when I was posted back to Singapore and Patsy was finally able to get some work doing relief jobs in civilian hospitals. Then, as my demobilisation was approaching, the Suez crisis suddenly blew up.

I was to be medical officer on a troop ship, a Norwegian passenger vessel commissioned by the army, but we were now faced with a serious dilemma: there was no place for Patsy. We had two iron trunks packed in our minute apartment in Singapore and Patsy was sitting weeping on one of the trunks because she had no idea how she would get home, or whether she would see me again after I had gone to meet the boat. I told her not to worry because I would do my best to get her on board one way or another.

As I arrived on the *Skaubryn,* a beautiful ship, I was met by a young German of about my age who turned out to be the ship's doctor. I told him of our problem and he was amazed that the British army would let one of its officers' wives languish abroad, with no provision for repatriation. He immediately took me to the captain, a tough Norwegian, who was indignant, sympathetic and decisive: he engaged my wife as the ship's nurse on the spot, and agreed to pay her one Norwegian crown a week.

I rushed back to the apartment and told Patsy that she had a job. We were overjoyed and the icing on the cake was that we were allotted one of the best staterooms on the boat.

Back Down to Earth

When we arrived six weeks later, at my parents' home in Epsom, I realised that I had to get a job.

In those days, training as a surgeon meant first obtaining two parts of the Fellowship of the Royal College of Surgeons: the first in anatomy, physiology and pathology; and the second in the theory of practical surgery. There was an 85 per cent failure rate among those trying for the first part and 75 per cent for the second, so the gates to the surgical profession were rather difficult to open. In order to pass the first part of the Fellowship, it was generally considered sensible to spend a year or more learning and teaching anatomy. I applied for anatomy jobs at Guy's and at every London teaching hospital that had an anatomy department. However, my applications were consistently rejected and I became thoroughly depressed. My brother Donald, who was an undergraduate studying medicine at Oxford, said that they had a staff crisis in the anatomy department there and I ought to come and speak to their professor.

In the department of human anatomy at Oxford the post of junior lecturer (or demonstrator, as it was called) was open for the coming year. The professor offered me this post on a salary of £250 per year, which was scarcely enough to stave off hunger. Nevertheless, we were delighted, and we rented a small apartment in North Oxford. Donald shared the rent and Patsy took a job at the Radcliffe Infirmary as a staff nurse. I needed to get down to my studies, having gone all the way to the East and back without opening my copy of *Gray's Anatomy.* I worked frantically but, to my extreme embarrassment, the medical students I met at Oxford knew more anatomy than I did. This was a violent stimulus to study harder, as was the fact that I had only one shot at the exam because of our poverty, so I worked day and night.

It was well known that we were likely to be asked detailed questions about ossification centres of the bones of the developing foetus – that is, the points within the bones where calcification starts. The development of each bone in the foetus starts at a specified time so that some bones develop earlier than others. This information is primarily used for forensic purposes and can easily be obtained from a book so we thought it was a waste of time learning it. It was rather like learning telephone numbers and Patsy would despair if I failed to give her a correct answer when she asked for the date of an ossification centre. She would quiz me on these details even on those rare occasions when we took a punt out on the river.

There was scarcely an anatomy question in *Gray's* that I couldn't answer, and after all that, when I came to London to take the test, the questions didn't seem to be as searching as those Patsy had asked me. At the end of the vivas I went up to the Grand Hall of the College of Surgeons at Lincoln's Inn Fields and the porter read out the numbers of those who had passed. I was very pleased to be through the first gate, and a few days later a letter came through the post saying that I had come first in the exam and would be awarded the Hallett Prize of £10.

We invited Sir Wilfred Le Gros Clarke, head of the anatomy department, and his wife to supper, and Patsy cooked them an excellent curry. We knew that Le Gros Clarke had spent his early years as a doctor in Borneo and liked Eastern food. The evening seemed to go reasonably well and Lady Le Gros Clarke smiled sweetly and turned to my wife and said how much she had enjoyed the curry and how she also found it a most useful dish with which to get rid of her scraps and leftovers. The last word was muffled in a slight cry as her husband kicked her under the table. The next morning I was summoned to his office. 'Your wife looks very thin,' he said. 'I am going to raise your salary to £450 a year.' So the curry dinner transformed our income, and I started to work for the Final Fellowship.

I stayed in my job at the anatomy department, but also started a concurrent post as an orthopaedic house surgeon at the prestigious Nuffield Orthopaedic Centre in the Wingfield Morris Hospital. At the Wingfield, I operated on a lady with bunions and the next morning I went to see her and asked how she was feeling. She said she was all right, then looked me over carefully and said, 'I know who you are. The last time I saw you, you were playing the ukulele in the street in downtown Singapore. I especially came to the Wingfield Morris for my bunion operation so that I would not be operated on by somebody like you.' She did, however, recover from her operation. I was a little hurt: I thought she might have had pleasant memories of my music-making in Singapore.

Family Life

From the time of our marriage in 1956 in Hong Kong to the present day Patsy has been a constant and enthusiastic helpmate in all aspects of my work – and equally ingenious in managing our home life despite the many difficulties that have arisen. We were childless for two and a half years after we were married and this resulted in the present of a dog to keep us company. Since then we have always had one or two dogs: indeed, visitors often seem to feel that we are part of the dog's family, rather than the other way round.

When our first child Jane was born, on 25 January 1958, we were living in a small flat in North Oxford. The people in the flat above disturbed us with the noise of their parties and this interfered with my studies, but we in turn disturbed our neighbours in the flat below with the noise of our child at night. When I started my job at the Wingfield Morris Hospital we decided to rent a bungalow in Headington which had been previously occupied by Harold Ellis, Professor of Surgery at Westminster Hospital who later taught anatomy at Guy's and St Thomas's Medical School. It was very cold and we couldn't afford proper heating, so the only warm place in the house was the airing cupboard. Here Jane was nurtured in her own private incubator, kept warm by the immersion heater.

Chapter Three
The Shoulders of Giants

One of the joys of living in a university town like Oxford is the chance to meet people outside one's own special field, and sit at the feet of great masters of science and the arts. So I was delighted when my brother told me that Peter Medawar, the transplantation immunology expert, was coming to give a general science lecture. The subject was tissue grafting – a reminder of that ward round at Guy's when my initial questions about the technique swiftly reached a dead end.

Peter Medawar and the Beginnings of Immunology

The lecture theatre was crammed full of students and graduates, a testimony to Medawar's celebrity in his field and his enormous power as a lecturer. The man stepped on to the platform, the buzz of chatter stilled, and he held the room spellbound with his brilliant oratory and extraordinary subject matter. Afterwards, a student asked if it was possible to apply the results of Medawar's research to the treatment of human patients. After a pause, Medawar said, 'Absolutely not.'

My brother and I argued about this into the early hours of the morning. I felt there must be an application to humans, while my brother said that, as Medawar was the world authority on the subject, it was likely that he was right. Medawar himself, of course, never worked with human patients.

As ever, however, my rebellious nature spurred me on. The next morning I asked Sir Wilfrid Le Gros Clarke's secretary if I could speak to him and she said I could have two minutes. I told Le Gros Clarke that I wanted to study transplantation of organs and, having heard this wonderful lecture by Professor Medawar and knowing that he was a personal friend, I wondered if he would be prepared to write a letter of introduction on my behalf so that I could do research with Medawar. Le Gros Clarke was not impressed. 'Professor Medawar is a very busy man,' he said. 'You go and learn how to repair hernias and don't bother him with such childish notions.' Once again I was summarily dismissed.

It will be fairly obvious by now that Medawar was my hero in the field of transplantation, a man of high intelligence and powerful presence, possessing a rapier-like intellect in debate and a generous and kindly personality. He was born in Petropolis, close to Rio de Janeiro in Brazil, his father Lebanese and his mother English. He came to school in England and thence to Oxford, where he distinguished himself academically and met and later married a fellow biology student, Jean, who was a source of inspiration and support throughout his life.

During the war Medawar became interested in the biology of skin grafting and started working with a Scottish plastic surgeon called Thomas Gibson. (Gibson was an extremely skilful pioneer of plastic surgery, and a leader in his field. His services were especially in demand for the burns casualties of the war.) Together, they embarked on a series of important experiments on rabbits, which showed conclusively for the first time that skin grafts, often used in plastic surgery, behaved quite differently, depending on the donor source. Thus, a graft from the same animal to another part of its body, known as an 'autograft', was accepted permanently and grew lush fur. However, a graft from another rabbit, known as an 'allograft', after initially behaving in the same way as the autograft for three to four days (by developing a blood supply), became unhealthy over the course of the next few days, then scarred and died. This process of deterioration was accompanied by mononuclear cells called lymphocytes and other white cells from the circulating blood infiltrating the graft.

The crucial experiment involved using the same animal that had rejected the allograft and transplanting another graft or 'second set' from the same donor. Medawar and Gibson found that the second allograft deteriorated without ever 'taking' at all. A third graft, from another donor, however, behaved as the first had done, initially developing a blood supply and then beginning to look unhealthy and deteriorating over seven to ten days.

What did this pattern show? Medawar and Gibson had demonstrated an immune reaction: if one graft is rejected, and a second set from the same source is rejected more swiftly, it shows that the animal has developed immunity to that source – but not to other sources. This finding had enormous relevance to the problem of transplant rejection, which is discussed more fully later.

Two young research workers came to join Medawar. Rupert Billingham had served in the Navy and now planned a career in zoology. Leslie Brent, the youngest of the three and just out of university, had emerged from a horrific background in Nazi Germany, where his whole family had been murdered. He had been brought up as an orphan refugee in England, but somehow managed to rise above this terrible, traumatic childhood.

Over the next few years I followed the work of Medawar and his team, which was as gripping as a good novel. In 1955 he and his colleagues tackled another central issue in the problem of transplant rejection. This involved differentiating between the two types of twins in cattle: identical or monozygotic (originating from one egg); and non-identical or dizygotic (originating from two separate eggs). There was a practical reason for this research. Dizygotic cattle twins are sterile 'freemartins', so there was a need for a method of sorting identical from non-identical. Medawar became involved in this work when he was contacted by the animal husbandry department at the Berkshire Agricultural Research Station. His curiosity was sparked because he was already working on twins, and skin grafting seemed to offer a simple solution. Identical twins ought to accept grafts from each other permanently as autografts, while non-identical twins, he believed, would reject each other's grafts.

But the experiments were disappointing: non-identical cattle twins appeared to accept the grafts in the same way as identical ones, contradicting the pattern of rules proposed by Medawar and Thomas Gibson.

Instead of shrugging their shoulders and dismissing the failed experiment as uninterpretable, Medawar and his colleagues studied the literature on cattle twinning and found that the American biologist Ray Owen had discovered a peculiarity in the anatomy and physiology of non-identical cattle twins. This was the fact that, unlike non-identical twins in most mammalian species, the blood of non-identical cattle twins mixes freely in the uterus – that is, blood from each twin circulates in the other. Normally all a human being's red blood cells are of the same group: A, B, AB or O. Cattle have similar blood groups, with the exception of non-identical twins, in which some red cells are the equivalent of group A in humans and others of group B, and both types circulate without harm in both cattle twins.

This information, together with their related experiments, led Medawar's team to make an extremely important speculation. Embryos, they knew, had undeveloped immune systems. Could the presentation of foreign tissue to an embryo therefore condition the developing immune system to see this tissue as its own, and accept it? As it happened, this speculation fitted well with predictions on the formation of the immune system and antibodies then being developed.

The stage was now set for the most important experiments ever in tissue transplantation. Medawar and his team injected cells from one strain of mouse into the embryos of another strain. When the embryos developed into adult mice, skin from the donor strain was grafted onto them – and, amazingly, it was accepted. They later found that they could get similar results more easily by injecting newborn mice rather than embryos.

The team called this phenomenon 'immunological tolerance'; it was long-lasting, and specific to the particular donor. A problem arose here which, like many in science, eventually opened up new vistas of knowledge. Some of the mice became ill: their fur became ruffled and they looked like runts. This condition was initially named 'runt disease', and was shown by Billingham and Brent to be the result of immunological action by the donated cells against the recipient – 'a graft versus host disease'. The implications of this finding were very important. Any method of manipulating the immune system would have to be looked at carefully to ensure that donated cells did not work against the recipient, as in an autoimmune disease such as rheumatoid arthritis where the patient's own rogue cells attack the patient's joints.

Many people have looked at the work of this brilliant trio – Medawar, Billingham and Brent – and wondered which of them initiated the ideas. I knew all three men and I imagine that Medawar was the leader in terms of knowledge and experience, and Billingham and Brent were the highly innovative and motivated workers. The interaction between the three produced a rare and powerful intellectual chemistry which resulted in a plethora of important advances in transplantation immunology.

Inevitably there were others involved in this burgeoning field of knowledge. Milan Hašek in Prague had studied parabiosis of chickens and ducks – that is, the joining of eggs containing developing embryos together so that blood flows between the two embryo chickens, much as it does between dizygotic cattle twins. Independently of Medawar and his colleagues but at around the same time, Hašek found that this resulted in skin graft acceptance between the animals. Living and working behind the Iron Curtain, the Czech laboured, however, under a then dogmatic approach to biology, influenced by the Soviet biologist Trofim Lysenko. Yet, amusingly, at a time of confrontation between the USSR and China Hašek made Muscovite and Peking ducks tolerant to each other! Nevertheless when Medawar heard of Hašek's work, he was quick to acknowledge it and the two became friends.

The Nature of Originality

It will be evident, from what I've written of Medawar and his partners in discovery, that they were highly original thinkers. In science, originality is regarded as the most important and precious attribute. Yet, at the height of his fame, Isaac Newton wrote to Robert Hooke, 'If I have seen further it is by standing on the shoulders of giants,' meaning that his advances depended upon the findings of previous scientific geniuses. Originality is, in any case, an elusive concept because new ideas rest on the foundations of past observations, and also on explanations which no longer fit and therefore fire the great innovators to discover the truth.

As David Horrobin wrote in the *British Medical Journal* in 1978:

> The greatest discoveries, the ones which change the direction of well-established disciplines, often occurred because of utterly irrational persistence (Erlich), following up of seemingly trivial observation (Fleming), or sacrilegious crossing of disciplinary lines (Pauling, with haemoglobin). Virtually never has a specialised researcher, well trained in a particular discipline, discovered anything of importance by pursuing a project thought reasonable by an expert committee. (And here we should not forget that it was probably Fleming who advised the MRC not to support on a large scale the penicillin work of Chain and Florey.)

The most important advances have been achieved by obsessively driven and curious individuals. Their motives are often mixed but usually involve the challenge, excitement and intense personal satisfaction of surmounting obstacles in order to achieve an objective.

Although virtually all science starts with an educated guess, or hypothesis, it is only the repeated successful testing of such a theory that qualifies it to join a body of knowledge that is accepted by most sane people. Thus, for example, an engine of sufficient thrust and an airframe of appropriate materials and configuration can be expected to fly, as witnessed by the successful air communications that we now take for granted. The same is true of the circulation of the blood, and the basic machinery of living matter, animal, plant, bacterial, fungal and viral.

This century has seen great leaps in our understanding of

biology. For instance, until the 1950s, we did not know how biological information was transferred from one generation to another. There seemed to be good evidence that all the data necessary to construct a living being lay in the nucleic acids of the fertilised egg, a fusion of the male sperm and the female ovum. But we did not understand how the basic information was transcribed. It was James Watson and Francis Crick's great discovery, that DNA is shaped like a double helix (a kind of twisted rope ladder), which led to the understanding of how this remarkable molecule stored the genetic code by which characteristics are handed down.

The collaborative work of Watson and Crick depended on the chemistry of two very different individuals who tossed their ideas back and forth and listened carefully to the signals of others working in the field, who inevitably were regarded not only as fellow scientists but as competitors. Reading Watson's account of their work in *The Double Helix*, one gains the impression that they were running a race, but they always acknowledged their debt to others, particularly Rosalin Franklin, whose painstaking and beautiful x-ray crystallography pictures were essential in constructing the model of the DNA molecule.

Overcoming Obstacles

Many important observations in the biological sciences have been established only after years of painstaking study, selection of evidence, disappointments and then worry on the part of the innovator as to how the new ideas would be received. In past centuries the Church was enormously powerful in enforcing religious dogma, and there were many instances of scientists suffering because their ideas contradicted the accepted religious teaching. Galileo Galilei, for instance, was lucky to escape serious punishment by the Inquisition in the early seventeenth century, while some decades later William Harvey, the great physician who produced the first treatise on the circulation of the blood, was vilified by many of his contemporaries because his views clashed with the classical explanations accepted by the Church. And Charles Darwin spent more than twenty years amassing a vast amount of data as ammunition against his expected critics, providing a new way of looking at evolution and the origin of species. Yet, even to this day, his theories cannot be taught in some countries.

The Church has not been the only enemy of scientists: sometimes doubt comes from within the scientific ranks. Joseph Lister, for example, experienced opposition from his colleagues in his advocacy of antiseptic surgery. And the Hungarian obstetrician Ignaz Semmelweis, working in Vienna, pointed out that doctors moving from the post mortem room directly to the delivery room resulted in an extremely high instance of fatal sepsis in women having babies. However, if the doctors washed their hands, the dreaded puerperal sepsis was usually avoided. Semmelweis was so ridiculed that he lost his job, yet there is now a statue of him in Vienna.

Fashion is also important in science and in recent years, following Watson and Crick's discovery, there has been a boom in molecular and cell biology advances. These subjects have been particularly popular because they shed light on the nature of cancer and, it is hoped, increase our understanding of HIV. Meanwhile the old-fashioned subject of anatomy has been devalued in intellectual circles, to such an extent that many departments of anatomy are headed by people who do not know even the elements of the structure of the human body and yet are responsible for teaching medical students. It is received wisdom that all gross anatomy has now been described, published and is available in books and so no new research is needed.

In the light of this, it is interesting that two personal friends of mine have both worked in the field for many years and made important advances in gross anatomy. The first, Paco Torrent Guasp, was a GP in the small Spanish town of Denia, near Valencia. He had long been interested in cardiology, and fascinated by the anatomy of the heart. Using a needle to tease out the fibres of an ox heart, he soon became convinced that the arrangement of the fibres was not as shown in the textbooks. In fact, the muscle fibres form a spiral. This explains why the heart, when it contracts, displays an easily observed twisting movement, and raises a number of important questions concerning the function and diseases of the heart, and surgical approaches to that organ.

Despite the importance of his discovery, as a small-town doctor Guasp had difficulty getting his observations published. Then, when a prominent foreign professor visited him in Denia, the man tried to publish Guasp's work as his own. Fortunately Guasp had friends with access to the more commonly cited journals and now his labours of more than forty years are recognised.

The second example is in orthopaedics. Forty years ago Harry Crock, a distinguished Australian spinal surgeon, started studying the blood vessels supplying the bony spine and the spinal cord. He found that the course of these small blood vessels in bones and their origin had not been examined in great depth because they were difficult to dissect, and were not regarded as particularly important. However, Harry Crock was well aware of the fact that many apparently splendid operations to rectify structural problems of the spine failed for biological reasons.

Most spinal surgery aimed at stabilising the vertebrae is based on the structural integrity of the bones, which form arches around the spinal cord, and are layered one upon the other like stones forming a column. This mechanical approach would be fine if one were building an inert spinal column, but bones are living structures, surviving and flourishing because of their blood supplies. Sticking a large screw into a bone without taking these blood vessels into account often leads to necrosis of the bone, loosening of the screws and the patient being worse off than before the operation. The same is true of the treatment of many fractures and replacement of joints where little attention had been paid to the blood supply and venous drainage of the part of the bone that was to receive the implant and the screws and cement.

After four decades of painstaking dissection of bones, removing their calcium and injecting the blood vessels, Harry Crock has produced his *magnum opus*: a most beautifully illustrated book like a modern version of the classic by Versalius, the great sixteenth-century anatomist. One hopes this knowledge will lead to a more intelligent use of screws, cement, metal and plastic plates in bones, in a way that will not interfere with the blood supply on which their life depends.

The Beginnings of Transplantation

Just as the Wright brothers' plane launched the science of aviation, so some advances in organ transplantation have changed our whole way of looking at medicine and have restored many patients facing death to an excellent quality of life for many years. This has depended on the work of different individuals all over the world, and their many contributions have helped us to deal with the two major problems involved in organ transplantation: the surgery and the immunology.

The donor organ must be alive and healthy when removed. Once its blood supply is stopped it will deteriorate, but this process can be slowed by cooling, using the domestic process of refrigeration. The donor organ must be transferred to the recipient in perfect condition and its blood supply restored, and if it has an essential duct such as the ureter, the bile duct or the bronchus, this has to be provided with free drainage. Fortunately, the best means of preserving the organ turned out to be the easiest to arrange, namely simple cooling with ice in an environment of fluid and electrolytes that will not harm the organ.

Since the beginning of the century when Alexis Carrel discovered a safe way to join arteries and veins by sewing the tubes together with silk, there were a number of attempts at kidney grafting both in animals and humans. Carrel himself, and later William Dempster in England and Morton Simonsen in Denmark, performed important experiments transplanting kidneys in dogs, showing that like skin autografts, they could work perfectly indefinitely, but allografts were rejected after 7-14 days. Xenografts, from other species, were destroyed immediately.

It was in Boston at Harvard Medical School and the Peter Bent Brigham Hospital that the first major advances of kidney grafting in man were made.

The Peter Bent Brigham Hospital was a unique and splendid institution, small and elite with high-powered research going on in every department. Each of these departments was part of Harvard Medical School, and it was a true university hospital. The department of medicine, under George Thorn, had an international reputation. One of its most important divisions, dealing with kidney disease, was headed by John Merrill, an enthusiastic and innovative doctor always prepared to listen to new ideas in order to obtain better treatment for his patients. Merrill was one of the first in North America to develop the dialysis technique invented by Dr William Kolff in the Netherlands during the Second World War, and the dialysis equipment constituted one of the most important factors enabling the Brigham to pioneer kidney transplantation.

Francis Moore, the Brigham's surgeon-in-chief, had been appointed to the prestigious Chair of Surgery of the hospital at the relatively tender age of thirty-four. He had had a brilliant academic career which took an intriguing turn when he treated burns patients after a fire at the Coconut Grove night club in Boston. This experience left Moore fascinated by the body's response to trauma, particularly injuries and surgery. His work has been extremely influential in improving the treatment of patients before and during major surgical operations. Moore was an unusual character – one of those people who seem to thrive on no sleep. In fact, he would often interview young surgeons and research workers at three or four in the morning.

Much work on vascular surgery – that is, to do with the arteries, veins and valves of the body – was taking place in Moore's department, and among the young surgeons two were especially important in the history of transplantation: Charlie Hufnagel and David Hume.

Hume was the chief of surgery at the Medical College of Virginia in Richmond, who with Charlie Zukoski had been working with 6MP when I was at the Royal Free. Hufnagel had designed a plastic ball and socket to replace defective valves in the aorta, the great artery issuing from the heart. This artificial valve made quite a loud clicking noise, and patients given the device were regarded as anti-social in cinemas and other quiet places because of this insistent internal clicking, however vital to their health. In Moore's department, Hufnagel worked with Hume on kidney transplantation techniques. And in the early 1950s a programme of kidney grafts for patients dying of kidney disease was established at the Brigham.

Francis Moore and George Thorn were the chiefs responsible for the surgical and medical services, while the operations were performed by Hume. The results of the kidney transplants in these patients were better than might have been expected from studies in skin grafts, and raised two important new issues. First, there was an apparent difference in the rejection of the kidney, a vascularised organ, and skin, which is primary non-vascularised tissue. Secondly, patients who were sick with the uraemia of kidney failure (in which urine cannot be passed and therefore accumulates in the blood) were less able to mount an immune reaction against a kidney graft.

Shortly after these kidney allograft attempts, a patient was sent to Merrill, the referring doctor, who laid the groundwork for the historic operation when he noted the remarkably valuable information – 'by the way, Richard Herrick is one of identical twins'. Richard Herrick, a twenty-three-year-old identical twin in the final stages of Bright's disease, came to the Brigham with his healthy twin, Ronald, who was prepared to donate a kidney. The operation, carried out on 23 December 1954 by Joseph Murray, was a complete success, and Herrick returned to work and led a normal life. Later he married and had a family. Murray was now personally involved in kidney transplant research, and he became chief of the new programme.

Interestingly, Murray had trained as a plastic surgeon, and later developed an international practice in the repair of damage to the skull and bones of the face. In the course of his training he had come into contact with research on skin grafting, which is, of course, an essential part of plastic surgery. The techniques of vascular surgery were also similar to many of the fine suturing methods needed in plastic surgery. Then, when he moved to the Brigham, he had become fascinated by kidney transplantation.

Murray's very meticulous, focused approach and attention to

detail were important factors in the success of his identical twin transplant programme. The programme became, in fact, a source of inspiration to all surgeons interested in organ transplantation, because Murray showed that if the surgery was performed swiftly and correctly, the transplanted organ would function perfectly, and indefinitely, provided that the donor twin did not have the same susceptibility to kidney disease from which the sick twin suffered. The good results he achieved with identical twins have stood the test of more than forty years.

Murray also became involved in the ethical and legal aspects of transplantation, especially when a pair of sixteen-year-old twin boys came to the Brigham for a kidney transplant. One suffered from irreversible end-stage kidney disease; the other was healthy. The potential donor was a minor, and by law could not consent to an operation that could apparently do him no good. The help of the law was sought and the case was presented to the Massachusetts Supreme Court in 1957. After lengthy deliberation, the learned judges' conclusion was that the operation should proceed with the parents' consent, since if deprived of the opportunity of saving the life of his brother, the healthy twin would be psychologically traumatised when he realised the implications of this in later life. The operation went ahead and was successful.

A man of deep religious convictions and generosity of spirit, Murray agonised over the ethics of transplantation, and always put himself in the position of the patient and considered the impact of the treatment on their family. I learnt a great deal from him in this respect. In 1990, Murray was to win the Nobel Prize for Medicine.

The second problem, preventing rejection of the organ when the donor is not an identical twin, was defined by Medawar and his colleagues, as already described. Gradually it became possible to overcome organ rejection in the laboratory and then in the clinic, using immunosuppression, initially with drugs used to treat cancer. More specific agents were found during routine screening in laboratories of substances produced by fungi and bacteria, but did not come into their own until many years later and will be covered in detail as the story unfolds.

Then, in the early 1960s, Michael Woodruff in Edinburgh and

Byron Waxman in the United States independently produced vaccines against the cells that cause rejection – lymphocytes – by injecting human lymphocytes into animals. The animals produced antibodies in the serum of their blood which could be used as vaccines against the lymphocytes that cause rejection. But it was difficult to purify these antibodies, and unwanted contaminants could harm the patient. This problem was addressed much later by two researchers in Cambridge, Caesar Milstein and Thomas Kohler, who were able to produce single pure antibodies in culture, each of which had only one target – a single molecule on the surface of a lymphocyte.

After the war, having experienced the horrors of Singapore's Changi Jail, Woodruff had been appointed to the Chair of Surgery in Dunedin in New Zealand. There he became interested in transplantation, performed tolerance experiments using rats, and described the phenomenon of 'graft adaptation' (whereby the graft changes its antigenic characteristics and develops resistance to rejection after being resident in a host).

It became apparent, from the work of Woodruff and others, that very powerful rodent anti-lymphocyte sera could be produced in rabbits. These sera were able to overcome the tendency to rejection, even in sensitised animals that had already rejected first set grafts. This unusual phenomenon was described by Medawar as 'erasing immunological memory'. Such a property, if applied to humans, would be extremely valuable, allowing us to treat many of the patients who have become sensitised by blood transfusions, pregnancies or previous grafts. Many of these patients have antibodies against most of the population and it is very difficult to find donor kidneys for them.

In 1957 Woodruff moved to the Chair of Surgery in Edinburgh and in 1960 he carried out a series of successful renal transplants. One recipient was a middle-aged man with an identical twin who donated a kidney. The recipient recovered well but six years later died (as did the donor twin) of stomach cancer. Woodruff also described the phenomenon of tolerance in non-identical human twins who had shared each other's blood circulations as embryos. This is very unusual in humans but, as Medawar had discovered, it is normal in non-identical cattle twins. At Edinburgh Woodruff continued studies of immunosuppression, obtaining improved anti-lymphocyte serum preparations, with reduced toxicity, which were effective in large animals.

These developments have made organ transplantation a reasonably successful therapy in the clinic, and so sought after by patients in need that there is now a serious shortage of organs for transplantation. This need is driving commercial institutions to undertake applied research on transplantation of organs from animals to humans, known as xenotransplantation. (Grafting organs from pigs to humans is surgically possible.) Huge pharmaceutical companies are the only institutions with sufficient financial resources to underwrite these extremely expensive experiments, and we do not even know at this stage whether or not the biological problem is soluble. However, research driven by a need is often successful in a remarkably short period of time.

All these factors – the needs of patients, the dedication, drive and curiosity of individual scientists, and the discoveries of those 'giants' who have gone before – combined to let us take the first few, vital steps in organ transplantation.

Chapter Four
Into the Unknown

In 1958, having learnt to do hernias as instructed by Wilfred Le Gros Clarke, I passed the final examination for Fellow of the Royal College of Surgeons, and therefore became entitled to apply for a job as a registrar in surgery. But my applications to most of the medical schools in London were rejected, and although I was sometimes shortlisted I would come home to Patsy in Epsom, where we were living with my parents, shaking my head, so that she knew before I spoke that I had failed yet again.

Finally I applied for a registrar's post at the Royal Free Hospital. The Royal Free Medical School had been founded to train women in medicine. Although by now the staff and students were mixed, women still predominated, and the hospital was not regarded as a first choice by most young surgeons. There was no academic department of surgery, although Professor Sheila Sherlock had just moved, like a tornado, from Hammersmith Hospital to the Royal Free and was establishing a medical liver unit of world renown.

Dogs in the Beds

I was surprised and delighted to be offered the job at the Royal Free interview. One of the interview panel was a newly appointed young surgeon, John Hopewell. He asked me if I had done any research, and I said, 'No, but I would like to work on organ transplantation.' He seemed to approve of this, and once I started working at the hospital he encouraged me to become involved in experimental work. At the time Hopewell was studying experimental transplantation of the ureter into the bowel of animals, since this was one of the methods used to treat cancer of the bladder in man. Urine draining into the bowel caused poorly understood metabolic changes that Hopewell was beginning to unravel.

Hopewell worked at the Buckston Browne Farm in Downe, Kent, which was one of the very few experimental laboratories in the country where large animals could be studied. It was part of the Royal College of Surgeons and adjacent to Charles Darwin's house. All of which was wonderful: but a serpent lurked in this experimental Eden. There was no money for me to do any research. Although Hopewell introduced me to David Slome, the Professor of Physiology of the Royal College of Surgeons, and Superintendent of Buckston Browne Farm, Slome unfortunately had no money to sponsor my research. Moreover, I had no chance of obtaining a grant, since I had a spectacular paucity of credentials.

Slome was, however, fascinated by the idea of organ grafting, and he allowed me to attempt to transplant kidneys in rats. At that time no successful technique for this procedure had been described, and I started using plastic stents – a kind of bridging tube – for the vascular junctions. After many hours late at night grappling with the technique, I eventually obtained kidney function in one of my experimental animals for twenty-four hours, but it seemed unlikely that I would progress any further.

One night, Slome came into the laboratory. He pointed out to me that I was persistently and constantly failing but, since he was convinced that I was keen, he would let me transplant a kidney in a dog. I had read about the technique of kidney transplantation in the neck, published independently by Morten Simonsen, a young physician working in Denmark, and William Dempster, a surgical researcher in Britain. Although Dempster was still in London, he was said to be rather unapproachable. I therefore did the transplant on my own, using an intra-abdominal technique very similar to that practised clinically today. I was untrained in vascular surgery and the facilities were very primitive: the surgical light was an Ovaltine tin fitted with an ordinary bulb. The head technician, Frank Watson, had worked with Dempster before he moved to Hammersmith Hospital and was very helpful. He gave me some guidance but I had to teach myself the technique.

Meanwhile, in our general surgical work at the Royal Free in London we admitted all kinds of patients, and one day I operated on a man with jaundice. Some three weeks later the house surgeon and I both became ill. The thought of food made me sick, I turned bright yellow and became extremely weak. My doctor diagnosed hepatitis and said he would send me to Professor Sheila Sherlock. However, I had seen the beautiful liver biopsy illustrations in Sherlock's book *Diseases of the Liver*, and I knew that her department was interested in collecting more specimens for research purposes, so I felt I would be safer at home looked after by my wife rather than have a large needle inserted into my liver. There was no specific treatment for hepatitis other than loving care, which would be superior at home.

Patsy was pregnant at the time and she was given gamma globulin injections to reduce the risk of her getting hepatitis. Every day I would look in the mirror and I seemed to be getting more jaundiced. This saddened me, as my work was going well and I wanted to finish it. Thankfully, after about six weeks I suddenly felt a desire for food and the jaundice started to wane. For a doctor, illness is an impartial and severe teacher – my hepatitis left me with more sympathy for all patients, but especially those with liver disease.

Eighteen months after Jane's birth, our second daughter, Sarah, arrived. At this time I was well again and very busy with clinical surgical commitments at the Royal Free, so I spent many hours on the road between the King's Cross branch of the Royal Free Hospital, and the Buckston Browne Farm in Kent. But it was difficult to maintain both an experimental and a clinical surgical interest, and although Hopewell was very supportive, my other chief, George Quist at the Royal Free, was not impressed with academic surgery. He warned the sister in the surgical ward to keep an eye out for me because he feared I might start filling the patients' beds with dogs!

I had a lucky start. My first attempt at kidney grafting in a dog was surgically successful as an autograft: the animal survived after I removed its other kidney, despite the fact that the operation had taken a very long time. Slome was pleased with this result although the next ten technical failures disappointed him and me. Eventually the technique was reasonably successful, and in the meantime I had studied the literature on transplantation. Amazingly, this could be done in a few weeks in 1959, whereas now it would be difficult to get through half the publications in a lifetime.

By far the most popular way of depressing the immune response at this time was by exposing the whole body to x-rays, and clinics had just started using this method – with disastrous results. X-irradiation does kill lymphocytes, but it also does away with other blood-forming cells, and it damages the bowel. There were only two successes from many attempts: the good results were between non-identical human twins, with one operation performed in Paris by Jean Hamburger's group and the other at the Peter Bent Brigham Hospital, part of Harvard Medical School in Boston.

Professor David Smithers generously gave me permission to use the new cobalt x-ray machine at the Surrey branch of the Royal Marsden Hospital, as long as I worked at night when the patients no longer needed it. My knowledge of gamma rays was rudimentary, however, and my practical experience nil. The senior technician in the cobalt unit showed me where the switches were, worked out the dose so I could start at eight o'clock in the evening, as long as I was out by eight o'clock in the morning, and then went home.

Patsy helped me with these experiments in the cobalt unit, anaesthetising dogs and giving slow irradiation, first on one side and then on the other. It was spooky and exhausting work, with the ever-present anxiety that you might accidentally fry yourself. X-irradiation of 900 rads to the whole body produced severe depletion of the bone marrow and all the white blood cells disappeared. The dogs nevertheless rejected their grafts aggressively, almost as quickly as unirradiated dogs. To increase the dose to supra-lethal levels and give bone marrow grafts was too drastic and had been tried in humans without success.

I began to wonder whether anti-cancer drugs might prove to be an alternative to x-irradiation. Ken Porter, then a junior pathologist at St Mary's in London, had worked at Peter Bent Brigham Hospital with Joseph Murray and had used Thiotepa, an anti-cancer drug, achieving some success with lengthening the life of skin grafts on rabbits. I therefore contacted Porter, who discussed his experiments and showed me a paper in that week's *Nature,* the science research journal, by two haematologists in the United States, Robert Schwartz and William Damashek. The two researchers had prevented rabbits from producing antibodies against human serum by treating them for two weeks with the anti-leukaemia drug, 6-Mercaptopurine (6MP). They also found that this effect persisted after the drug treatment had stopped. The animals were able to react normally against a different protein, bovine gamma globulin, a blood product from cattle. Ken Porter and I felt this was a much more promising approach than x-irradiation. We decided we would each investigate 6MP. He would study its effects on skin grafts in rabbits and I would see if it could prolong kidney allografts in dogs.

I started these experiments in the summer of 1959 and I was pleased to note that some of the dogs lived for longer periods with kidney grafts. Frank Watson, senior technician at Buckston Browne Farm, was particularly impressed, since he had seen several hundred kidney grafts performed by Dempster, and none had functioned as long as the grafts in the dogs treated with 6MP. When it was clear that the drug was an interesting compound, I telephoned Porter, but before I could give him my news he said, 'You remember the 6-Mercaptopurine experiments? Well, I tried it and there was no significant effect on rabbit skin allografts so I wouldn't bother to try it in a dog.' I was pleased that I had not heard this earlier, or I might not have attempted it. It was the first clear indication to me of how different tissues and species react to rejection.

I wrote a short paper on my dog experiments, and it was published in the prestigious medical journal, the *Lancet*, in 1960. Dempster wrote a strange letter to the *Lancet* in response, which seemed to indicate that he was sceptical of my results. This caused me distress, since it was my first scientific paper, and I was in a very junior position. But I soon had an opportunity to discuss my work with Michael Woodruff, the British pioneer in organ grafting, in Edinburgh. He was encouraging and thought I ought to contact Medawar, so, despite having been warned about how busy he was, I telephoned his secretary, very meekly asking if I might have a chance to speak to him. She said, 'I'll put you through,' and suddenly I found myself speaking to the great man himself. He gave me the impression that he had all the time in the world to talk, and invited me to a colloquium to be held at University College, London, on the state of the art of tissue transplantation.

My introduction to the world of biological science was a revelation. I met Peter Gorer, Avrin Mitchison and Leslie Brent, all destined to become international figures in the biology of transplantation, and was amazed at how generous and friendly the atmosphere and discourse were, even when there was strong disagreement. The open-mindedness and lack of dogma were in marked contrast to the hierarchical system of surgery.

My experiments meanwhile seemed to be sparking interest among other experts. I had a letter from Charlie Zukoski saying that he, working with David Hume, the chief of surgery at the Medical College of Virginia in Richmond, in the United States, had obtained results similar to mine with 6MP, although they had had trouble with toxicity and dosage. Hopewell was also delighted with my work and agreed to use the drug in clinical transplantation of kidneys.

Our First Kidney Transplant

Kidney transplantation was still in its infancy around the start of the 1960s. At that time it had yet to be performed at the Royal

Free, and dialysis – the artificial filtering of blood to take the place of lost kidney function – was only just being set up there by Hopewell and Stanley Shaldon.

But why were kidneys chosen as the first organ for transplants? As you will recall from the case of Jonathan in Chapter One, fatal kidney disease often used to afflict the young. When invading bacteria called streptococci caused a sore throat or an attack of scarlet fever, the patient sometimes produced a rogue antibody in response that attacked the kidneys. A condition called glomerolonephritis, or Bright's disease, would then set in and destroy the kidneys.

Of course, we cannot survive without these compact super-filters that lie in our flanks, mirror images of each other. Or at least, we *can* survive as long as one remains intact. As many people know, if one of two normal kidneys is removed, the other rapidly enlarges to do the work of two: maintaining the correct balance of water and salts in the blood; excreting poisons and waste matter; and manufacturing a protein which the bone marrow needs in order to produce red blood cells.

Our first kidney transplant at the Royal Free was planned in October 1959. Since I had performed many experimental kidney grafts, it was decided that I would operate on the person receiving the kidney, and John Hopewell would remove the kidney from the deceased donor.

The fifty-year-old woman who was to receive the kidney was gravely ill with polycystic kidney disease, in which the entire organ is full of cysts that stop it functioning as a filter. The disease is always fatal. The donor had had a fatal brain haemorrhage but was connected up to a ventilator, so her heartbeat continued only because her lungs were being mechanically inflated. Her family understood that this maintenance of heartbeat in their dead relative should be stopped, and generously gave permission for a kidney to be removed and used for grafting.

The ventilator was disconnected, and soon afterwards the donor's heartbeat ceased. Meanwhile the recipient had been anaesthetised. Then Hopewell started to remove the kidney while I simultaneously prepared the woman to receive it. I was just about to make an incision in the lower abdomen, when Hopewell appeared at the door of the operating theatre with a large bowl in his hands.

He was in an operating gown, but his mask was off and his face was a mixture of horror, disappointment and incredulity. His expression was so final and dramatic that it has often haunted me since. Without his saying a word, I knew something dreadful had happened. Out of the bowl Hopewell took first one kidney and then the other, both huge and deformed, with a multitude of small and large cysts. The donor had the same polycystic disease as the recipient!

The chances of this coincidence, we later thought, must be less than one in a million. But in fact, when we researched the literature, we discovered that haemorrhage from a ruptured artery in the space surrounding the brain is a particular hazard in patients with polycystic kidney disease, making the chances of finding diseased kidneys in a victim of a brain haemorrhage, although unlikely, not insignificant. Now, of course, we always check the kidneys first in similar potential donors.

It was awful to face the fact, but our first attempt was a serious setback. The recipient died of her condition, and we realised that a sound infrastructure was necessary if kidney grafting was to become established. We needed access to regular dialysis, and collaboration with colleagues in renal medicine, haematology, biochemistry, radiology and bacteriology, besides surgery and drugs to prevent rejection. And over the passage of time, it transpired that organ grafting was not cursed, but was simply more complicated than we at first thought. We had learnt the hard way – by failure.

Chapter Five

New Horizons

After the awful shock and disappointment of our tragic first attempt at kidney transplantation using 6-Mercaptopurine (6MP), I felt that I should work on transplantation research full time instead of part time in a busy clinical job.

Our first initially successful kidney transplant was carried out at the Royal Free, after I had left, by John Hopewell. The patient was a youth of seventeen who was transplanted in July 1960 but died forty-nine days later. He was the first patient to be treated with chemical immunosuppression, in the form of 6MP.

Experimental work was now, in fact, central to my aims, although it was always arduous and chancy. I'd had enough experience of it to realise that asking a question was not difficult, but for the question to be relevant, insight and luck were needed. Moreover, the experiments required to test a hypothesis had to be carefully thought out and executed meticulously in order to avoid mistakes. It is also possible to perform difficult and expensive experiments that turn out to be irrelevant to the question being asked, even when conducted accurately and interpreted correctly.

There are other problems. When a meaningful observation is made, it is quite likely that it won't be believed by the scientific community until it has been repeated by others. If the work has been done in Europe, Americans probably will not have heard of it unless it has been published in an international journal. If published in a language other than English, it will almost certainly have been passed over by the large English-speaking community of scientists. The most important contributions of the French to clinical kidney transplantation have been seriously undervalued for this reason.

For example, Professor Jean Hamburger, whom I mentioned in the previous chapter, was a most respected expert on nephrology at the Necker Hospital in Paris, where he established a famous unit. He was a physician of great integrity who felt that organ transplantation must be the future for treatment of patients in the final stages of kidney disease. Although his unit was highly innovative, it has often received rather scant credit in accounts of the early history of transplantation. The French have always been pioneers in surgery, yet Hamburger saw surgeons very much as technicians brought in to 'mend the pipes'. He wanted the best technicians to do a superb job but the intellectual aspects were for the physicians. Nevertheless he graciously invited me to Paris in 1960 to give a talk on 6MP as an immunosuppressant.

This was a fantastic experience for a young surgical registrar. Hamburger put me up in his house and I was treated with the utmost hospitality and friendliness. He knew that I was visiting a rival institution headed by the surgeon René Kuss, and he told me that he didn't really know what was going on there but if I could obtain any information, he would be delighted if I were to share it! Hamburger was a world leader in transplantation and collaborated with Jean Dausset, the Nobel Laureate, who was the first to describe and define human tissue groups.

In contrast to the deeply philosophical physician Jean Hamburger, Kuss was a practising surgeon renowned for his technical excellence and debonair attitude. He also received me generously and asked about the results obtained by Hamburger's group! It was very interesting for me to discover that in the city of Paris, where there were two world-class pioneers in organ transplantation, the rivalry between them prevented the sharing of information.

Kuss specialised in urology. He did some of the earliest kidney transplants and described the technique of transplanting the kidney in the pelvis. This technique was used by Joseph Murray at the Peter Bent Brigham Hospital in twin transplants and is a standard method still practised today.

Kuss's interests extended beyond medicine. His father (who was also a surgeon) had been a collector of Impressionist art when these paintings could be purchased for a few francs. And Kuss was also a collector and connoisseur of paintings. Visiting his apartment was like going to an art gallery and I was astounded by the originals that were hanging on his walls.

Research was the driving force for Kuss and Hamburger, however, and both worked for long years pursuing it. This is another important consideration for anyone engaged in scientific research: the number of experiments that need to be performed before a theory can be perceived as proven. Today, more and more powerful statistical evidence is demanded, yet many of the greatest scientific discoveries of the past have rested on a small number of observations made by an astute investigator, without any statistical analysis. And many experiments may have to be conducted to get statistical significance – a process that is not only time consuming but also extremely expensive, which is problematic when money for research has always been difficult to come by.

However, at this point, I was driven by curiosity and remained undeterred by such concerns. To do a full-time research job I had to find a suitable laboratory and financial support. I was concerned about the career implications of disappearing into a lab for a year or more: would I lose my place on the promotions ladder? Nevertheless, I felt that I had made an exciting observation – that drugs could prolong kidney graft survival – so I set off on this path.

Off to America

Given the gravity of my decision, and the need to choose wisely, I sought Peter Medawar's advice. He was extremely helpful, and agreed that, in order to get suitable funding, it would be sensible to go to an American laboratory. Knowing that I wished to become a clinician, he kindly wrote on my behalf to Francis Moore, head of surgery at the Peter Bent Brigham Hospital, part of Harvard Medical School, to see if I could get a post in his department to work under Joseph Murray.

I applied for funding and was fortunate enough to be awarded a Harkness travelling fellowship. The Harkness Foundation is an American philanthropic institution which at that time awarded travelling scholarships to the US for British and Commonwealth scholars in all disciplines. The Foundation took a paternal interest in the work and living conditions of those awarded the grants, and insisted they spent at least three months travelling around the US to understand the enormous size and variety of the country and so avoid the unbalanced impressions that merely working at one institution would encourage. A car was provided for these three-month excursions.

So, very excited, if a little fearful about job prospects for the future, Patsy and I set sail with Jane and Sarah (aged two and one) on the *Queen Elizabeth*. (Our dog went to live with my parents in Epsom.) After an enjoyable trip we docked in New York in a heatwave, and Customs were very aggressive and made us unpack every piece of luggage. Eventually they let us through and we were met by a representative of the Harkness Foundation, who conducted us to a little hotel where life was punctuated by the wailing of fire engines, police-cars and ambulances, which Jane thought were babies crying.

When I had started working with 6MP in London, I had been in contact by post with George Hitchings and Trudy Elion, doctors at the Burroughs Wellcome laboratories in New York, and they had invited me to discuss future compounds with them when I came to the United States. I took a little train to Tucahoe in the suburbs of New York City, and was received with great friendliness by these two great scientists, who were to receive the Nobel Prize for Medicine in 1989.

Hitchings and Elion had synthesised purine and pyrimidine analogues designed especially for the treatment of cancer. (Purines and pyrimidines are the two types of chemicals that make up DNA.) In the hope of finding a compound that was safer and more effective than 6MP, they gave me a number of these purine and pyrimidine analogues to investigate. With these in my brief-case I arrived at the Peter Bent Brigham Hospital, to be met by Murray, who was to be my immediate chief. Murray was about to go on holiday, but with typical American generosity offered me the use of his car and said he was delighted that I had come, and that I could join their irradiation programme.

This was an unexpected development and I was dismayed: I had hoped to test the drugs that Hitchings and Elion had given me on dogs. I explained to Murray that I had come to work in his department hoping to avoid the use of irradiation. I had, after all, had enough of the method at the Royal Marsden. To my relief, he said I could start with the drugs, and then, if they did not work out, I could join the irradiation programme.

I worked day and night, operating and taking care of my animals. Patsy helped me exercise and feed the dogs with excellent meals from the Brigham Hospital kitchen, better than we were able to afford for ourselves. The success of the drug treatment was monitored by testing the dogs' urine. Catching urine from the male dogs was easy, but from the females it required intense observation, then a rapid lunge to place the bowl on the grass in time. This manoeuvre became known to my colleagues as the 'Calne crouch'.

After his return from holiday, I was able to show Murray dogs with kidney grafts treated with 6MP who were doing well, and as soon as he saw them, he devoted a great deal of time and enthusiasm to supporting my work. BW57-322, an analogue of 6MP, later known as azathioprine or Imuran, seemed to be the best of these agents, a little superior to 6MP. The high point of these experiments was the presentation at the Brigham of the first canine patient to survive a kidney graft, treated with azathioprine, with normal kidney function at six months. After the case history had been read, the door was opened and my dog Lollipop pranced into the crowded auditorium, making friends with the distinguished professors in the front row. Soon after, the use of thiopurines in clinical transplantation enabled the first phase of clinical organ transplantation to be established, with moderate success.

Francis Moore was the father figure in all this work at the Peter Bent Brigham Hospital, and he himself decided to investigate liver transplantation in animals. Transplanting the liver is a formidable operation, and it was found that dogs would not survive it when the main vein to the liver and the main vein in the body, the vena cava, were clamped. So Moore devised a method of bypassing the blood by shunting it back to the heart via a system of tubes, and was able to obtain successful experimental liver grafts. However, he then found that they were rejected in much the same way as kidneys.

These studies were already going on when I arrived at the Brigham, and although I did not participate in the liver transplant experiments, I was familiar with the procedure and attended the conferences that were held on liver transplantation. It was an inspiring atmosphere. I was impressed by Moore's incisive logic and quick understanding. He encouraged debate among members of the department, even the most junior like myself, and in this environment it was possible to have a constructive dialogue between senior and junior staff without any fear of getting into trouble for expressing views that were contrary to those of the professor.

In addition to the kidney transplant experiments that I had commenced as soon as I arrived, I was also investigating techniques of heart and lung transplantation, which meant I had to stay overnight with the unconscious animal, lying next to it on a straw bed. I woke one morning with my arms and legs covered in enormous blood-filled ticks.

Things changed much for the better a few months after I started: new laboratories were fitted out, and from then on the facilities were excellent and the animal care greatly improved.

By this time my experimental kidney grafting in dogs was going well, and both Murray and Moore felt that this line of study should be encouraged. They gave me three technicians and no financial constraints on the amount of work done – *carte blanche*, in short, to pursue the work in exactly the way I wished. This was an opportunity that never could have occurred in Britain.

Meetings with Remarkable Surgeons

Throughout our one and a half years in America the children flourished. Patsy and I worked very hard, she looking after me, the children and the huge rambling house in Wellesley Hills belonging to an elderly engineer, while I consolidated the experimental programme I had begun in England. When my happy and fruitful fifteen months at Harvard Medical School came to an end, the time came for us to set off on our three-month tour of the United States, as stipulated by the Harkness Foundation. The Foundation itself provided a car, Murray lent me his tent and camping equipment, and off we set, on a camping jaunt that was to cover 15,000 miles.

It was a wonderful experience. Moore had kindly written to a number of his friends who were prominent surgeons in institutions along our route. We would arrive at a campsite, light a fire, cook our meal, sleep in a tent, and the next morning I would put on my suit and visit the university hospital nearby, usually giving a talk on my work on immunosuppression. Then back to the camp, and on to the next.

The children seemed perfectly suited to this peripatetic existence. They were healthy and happy and loved cooking on a camping stove, sleeping in a tent, and the outdoor life in general. I had been worried that one of them would get ill but the only person who succumbed was myself, developing some weird virus infection in Texas.

We had marvellous moments. In New Orleans we encountered a terrible rainstorm when camping near Lake Pontchartrain. The tent was on a slope, and water began to flood into it. We crouched at the relatively dry end until, fortunately, the water receded. The next day we drove 200 miles into Texas, and when we unfolded the tent a frog jumped out. I hope he was able to find a mate: the journey from Louisiana to Texas must have left him severely disoriented.

One of the most important visits I made on this trip was to David Hume, who had by this time moved from the Brigham to Richmond, Virginia, where he held the Chair of Surgery at the Medical College of Virginia. Hume was a charismatic person with enormous energy but a relaxed approach. He had worked like a demon on kidney transplantation at the Brigham; now his success in helping patients survive who would otherwise have perished brought him friends in what had previously been a hostile environment, since he was a 'damned Yankee' working in the deep South. He pursued kidney grafting with dedicated enthusiasm. He also had a number of outside interests, particularly flying, and his attitude to it was similar to his approach to surgery – that nothing was impossible.

Hume's work on kidney transplantation brought him into contact with other practitioners in the field, among the most eminent of whom was Thomas Starzl. At this time Starzl was transplanting kidneys from the inmates of penitentiaries, while Hume was transplanting from cadavers, and with two such powerful and forthright characters in the room, inevitably there were verbal clashes, which were much appreciated by Starzl's and Hume's surgical colleagues. At one scientific symposium the two attended, the debate swung back and forth and Hume asked his audience, 'Would you rather be an organ donor prisoner in Denver, or a brain-dead donor in Richmond?' The point became an important focus of debate for years afterwards – was it justifiable to use living organ donors? And if one used dead donors, how could one be sure that they were really dead?

Hume had immense charm and a generous disposition, and certainly would have continued to pioneer new areas in transplantation. He was already interested in liver grafting, and xenografting, or the grafting of organs from other species into humans. But it was not to be. About to travel back from a meeting in Los Angeles in a hired plane, he heard that the weather had deteriorated, and that it was unsafe to fly over the Rocky Mountains. He ignored this advice. The plane was caught up in a storm and crashed, and Hume was tragically killed in the prime of his surgical career.

The two other professionally interesting visits on this epic journey were to Stanford University in California and Seattle, Washington. At Stanford, Norman Shumway had, together with Richard Lower, developed a technique of transplanting hearts in

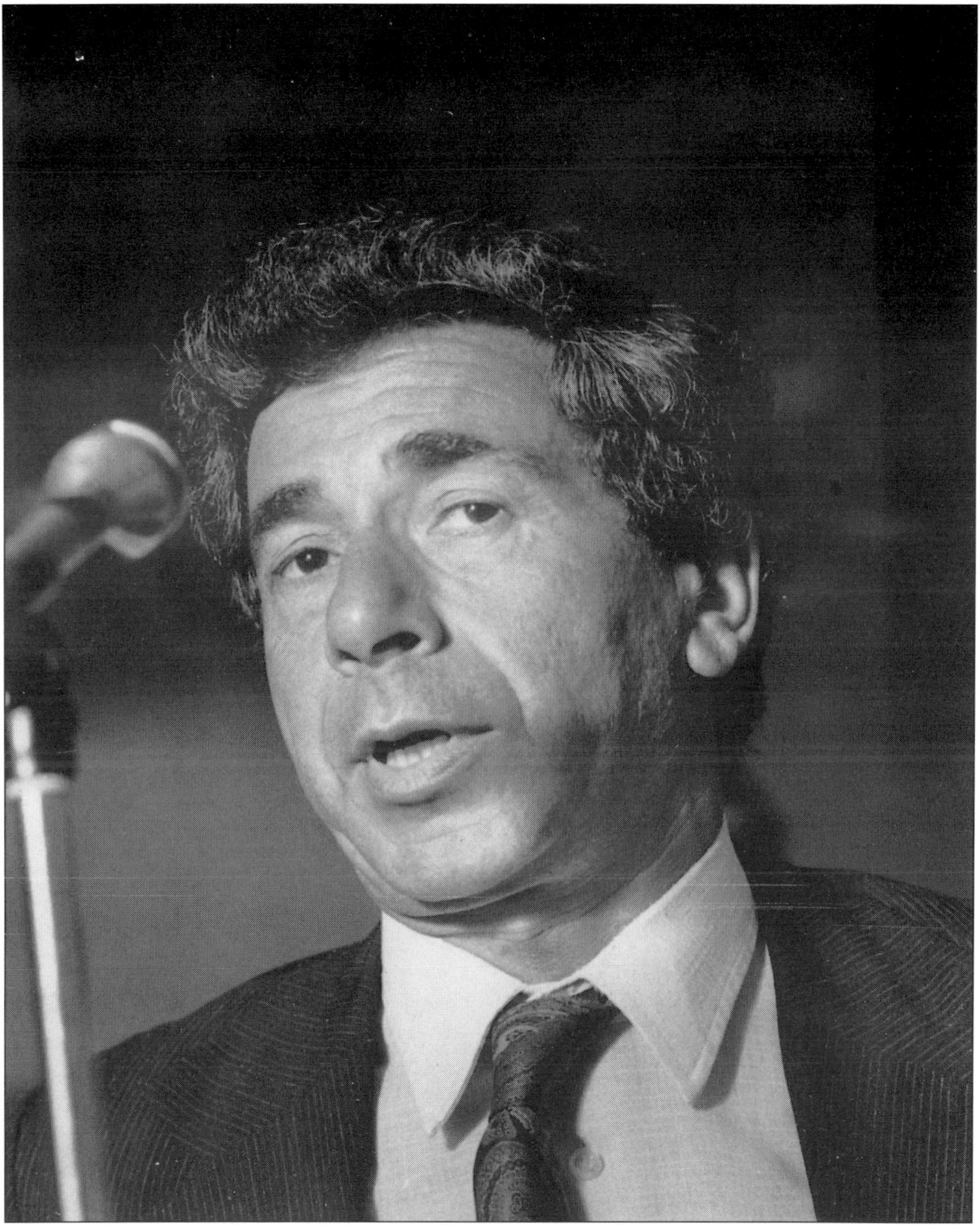

Giving lectures and addressing specialist conferences are very much part of my work (*Ted Polumbaum*)

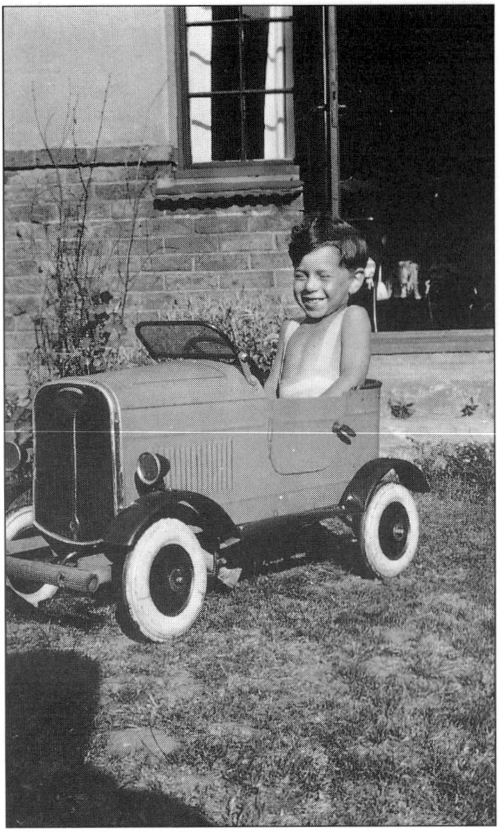

From an early age I was interested in mechanics and how things worked; this little car was a favourite toy

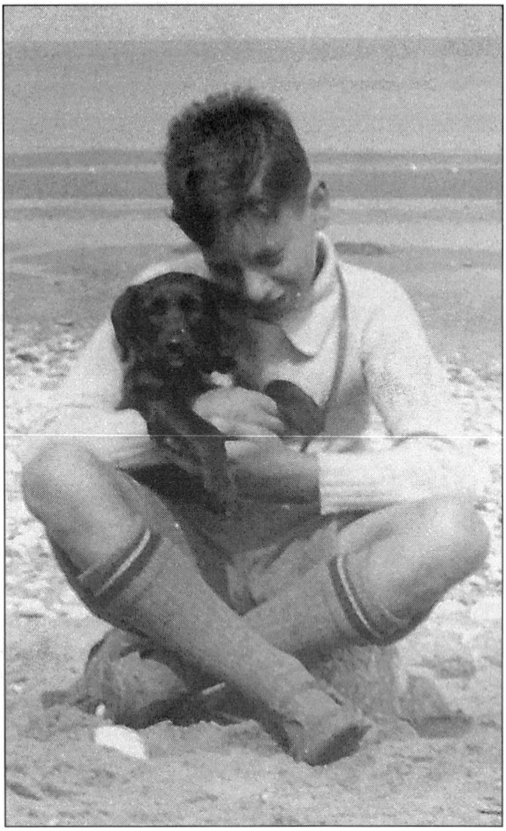

With a beloved pet Whisky, on a family holiday

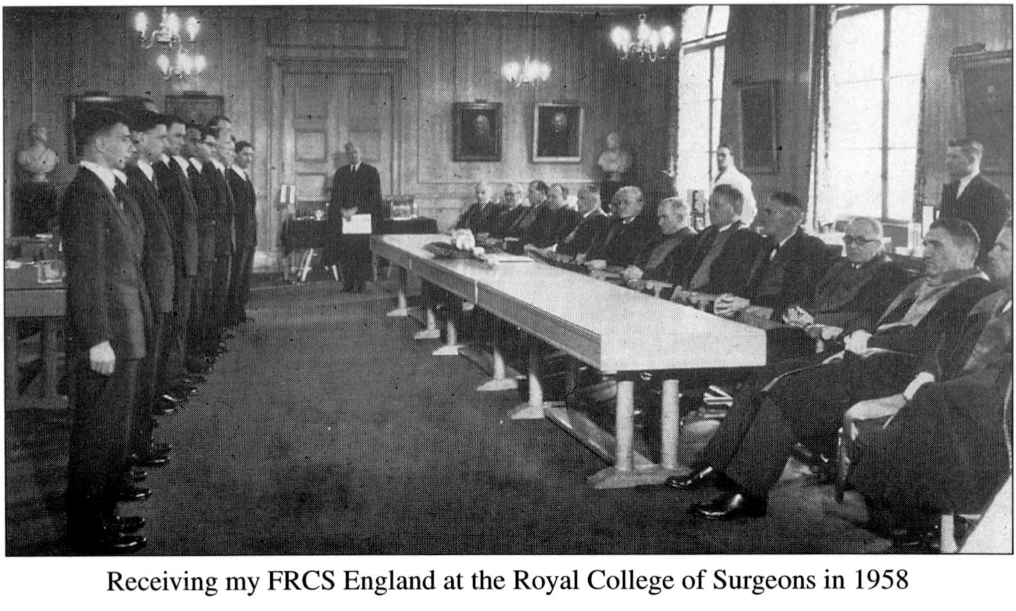

Receiving my FRCS England at the Royal College of Surgeons in 1958

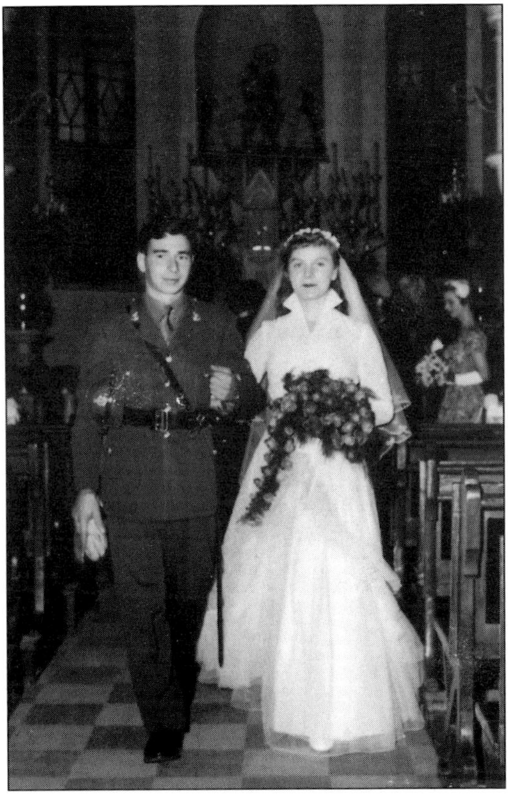

My wedding to Patsy in Hong Kong on 2 March 1956

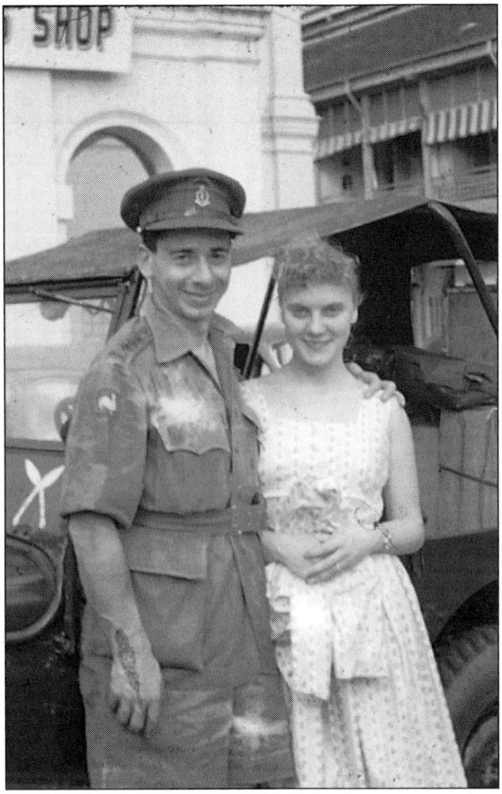

With Patsy, shortly after we arrived in Singapore later that month

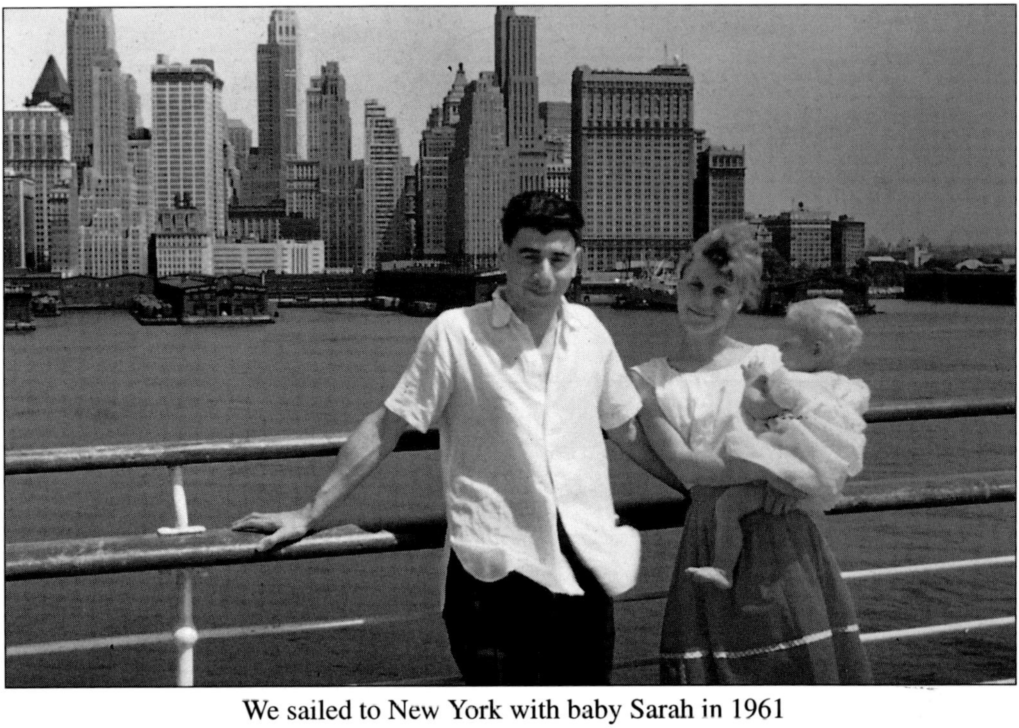

We sailed to New York with baby Sarah in 1961

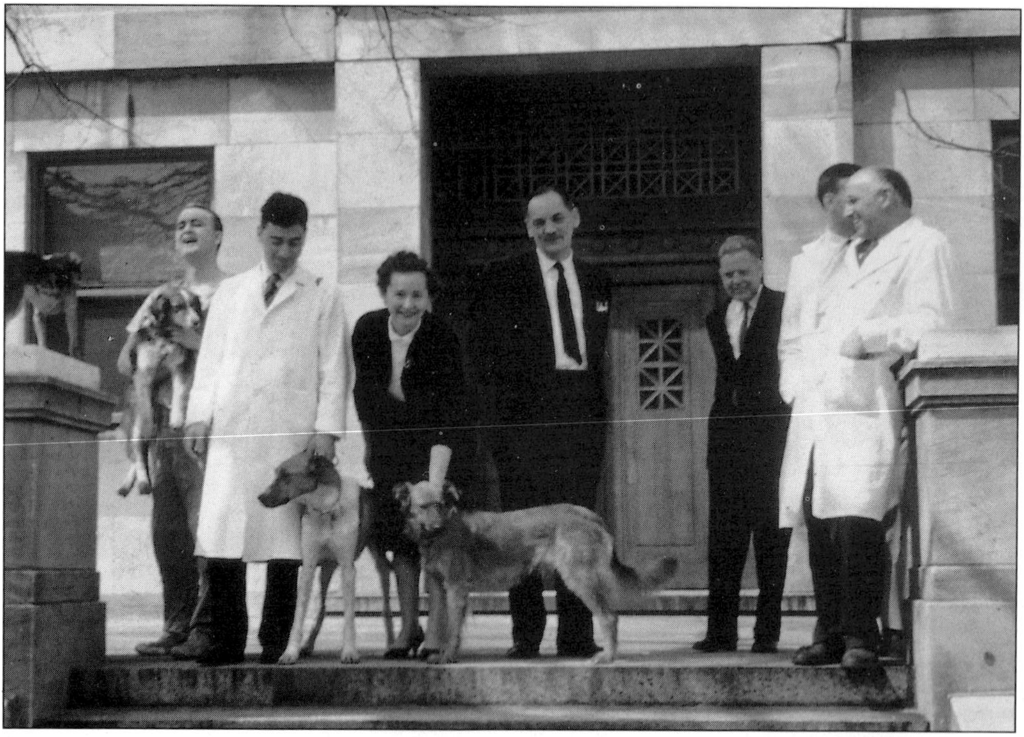

At Peter Bent Brigham Hospital, part of Harvard Medical School, with three Nobel prize winners: Dr Gertrude Elion, Dr George Hitchings (*4th from left*) and Dr Joseph Murray (*far right*) in 1961

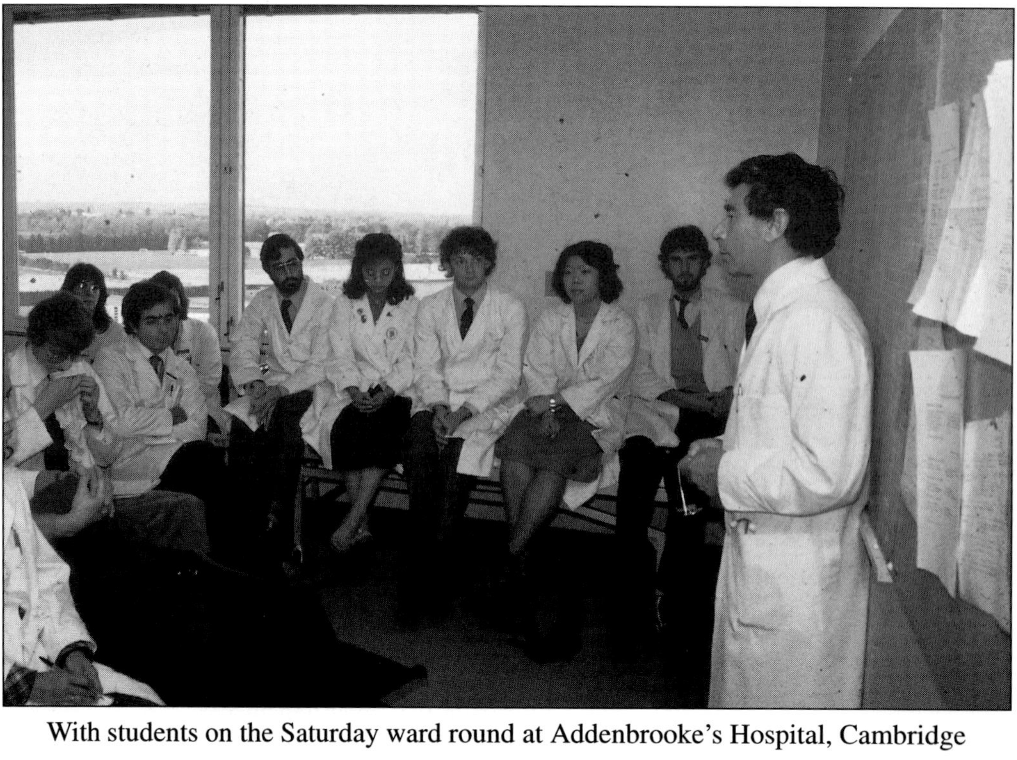

With students on the Saturday ward round at Addenbrooke's Hospital, Cambridge

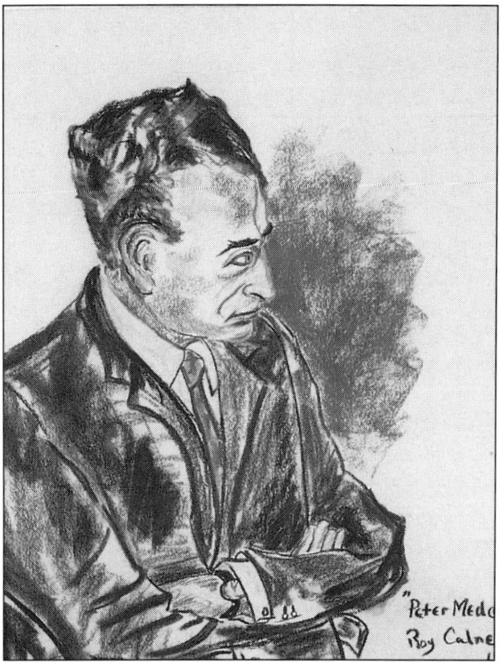

My paintings of four inspirational men: Sir Peter Medawar, the father of transplantation immunology

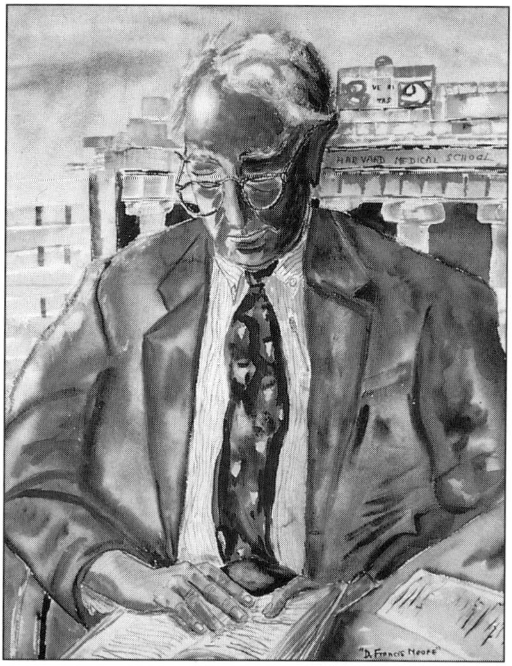

Dr Francis Moore, Surgeon-in-Chief at Peter Bent Brigham Hospital and pioneer in liver transplantation

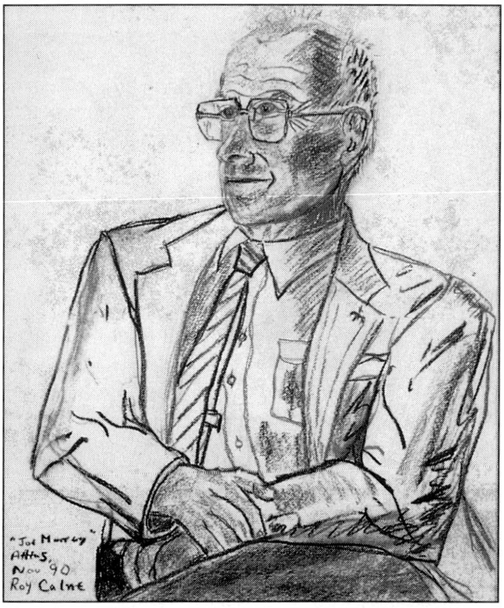

Nobel prize winner Dr Joseph Murray who undertook the first identical twin transplants in Boston

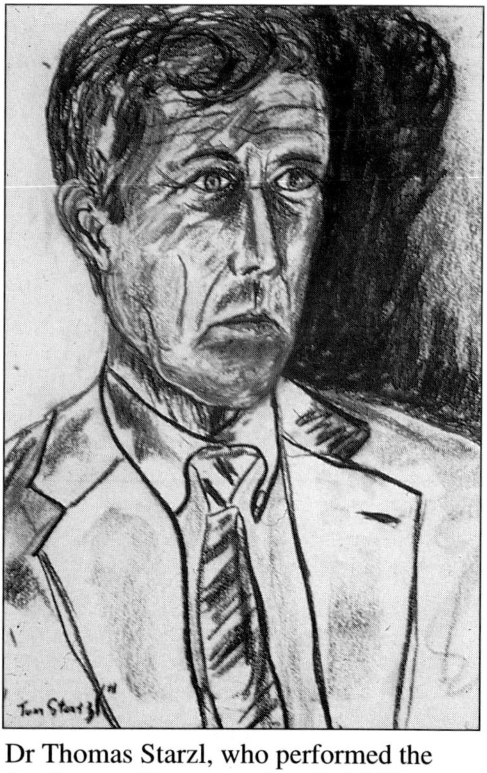

Dr Thomas Starzl, who performed the first human liver transplant in 1963

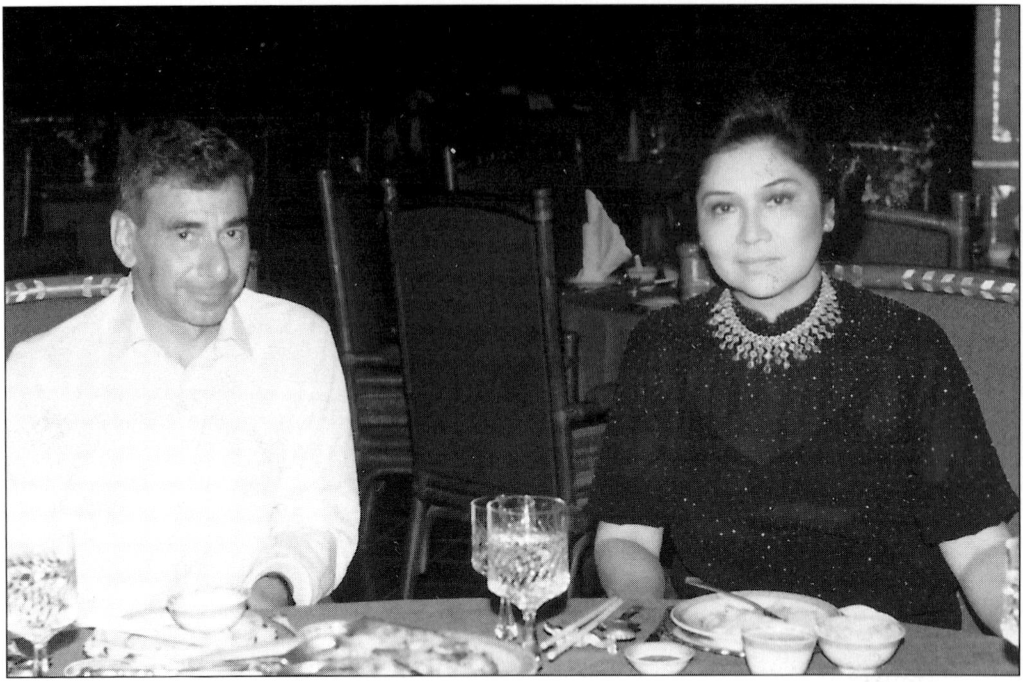

I was summoned to dinner with Imelda Marcos in Manila to discuss her husband's kidney transplant

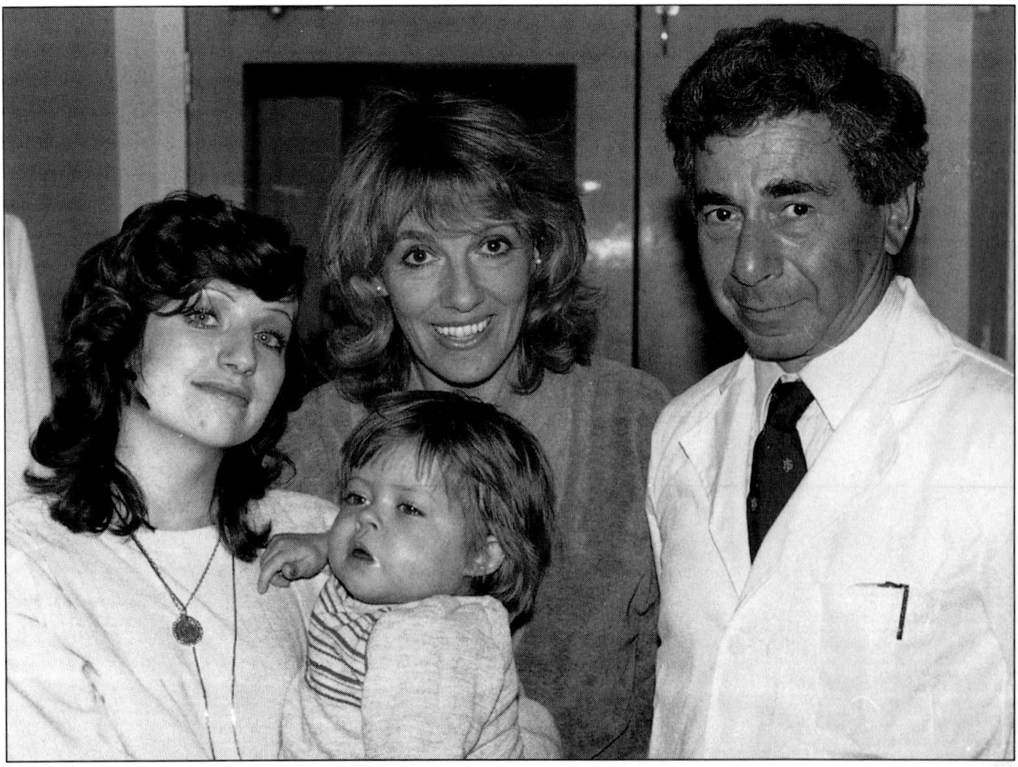

With Debbie Hardwick, her son Ben – the first child in the UK to have a liver transplant – and Esther Rantzen who had campaigned on his behalf (*Sunday Mirror*)

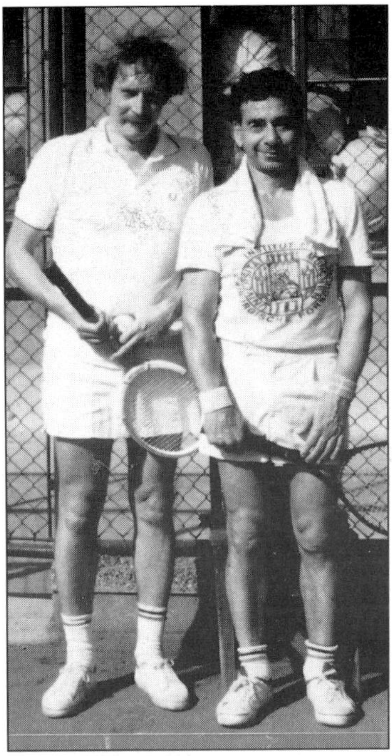

My recreations are tennis – here with Mike Lindop in the Jing-Jaing Club in Shanghai, China...

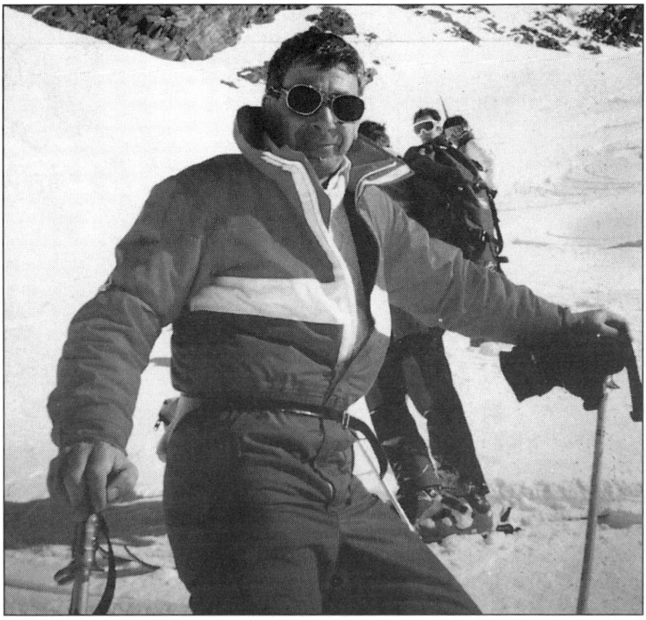

... skiing...

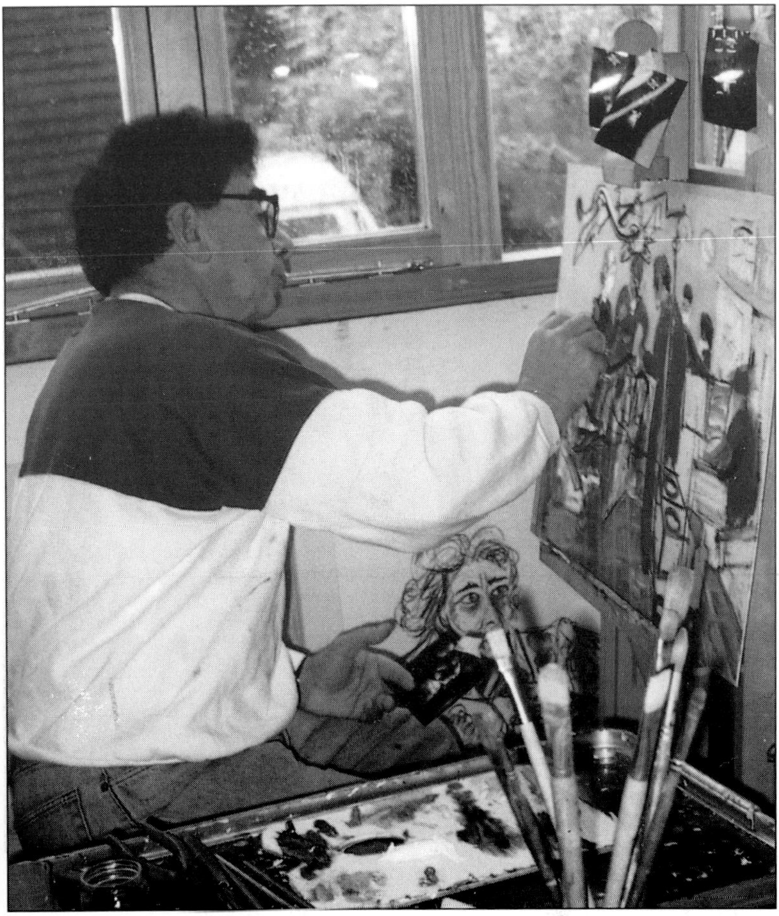

... and painting, in my studio at home

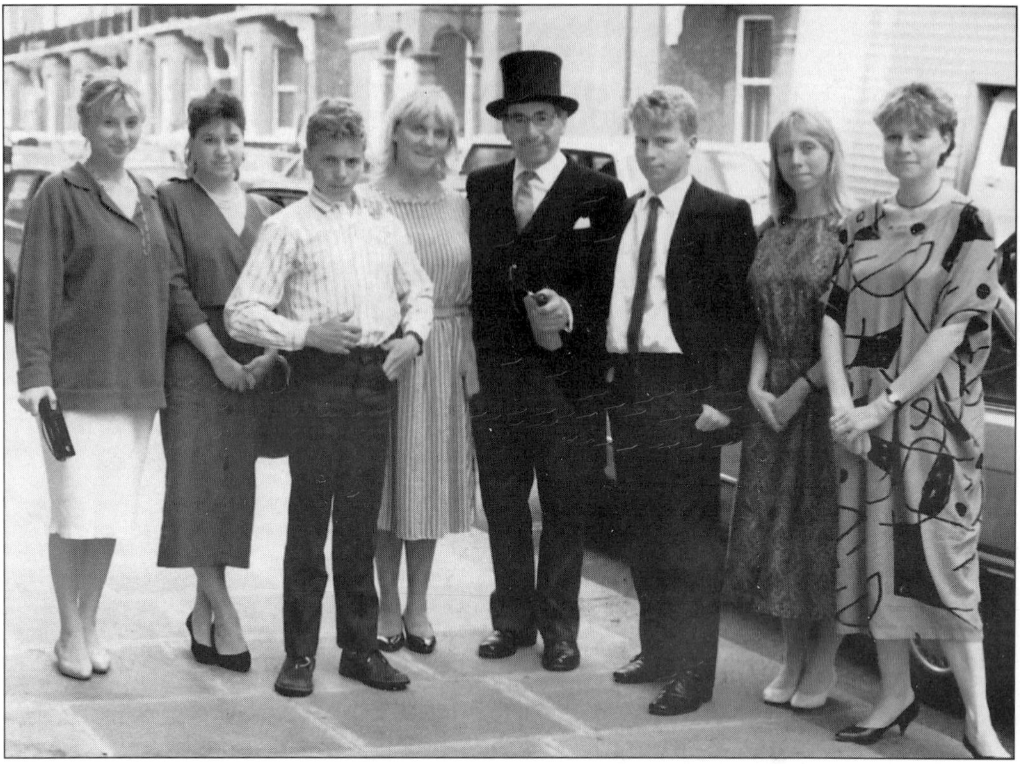

I was honoured with a knighthood in 1986. The whole family came to the investiture: *l to r* Suzanne, Deborah, Richard, Patsy, me, Russell, Jane and Sarah

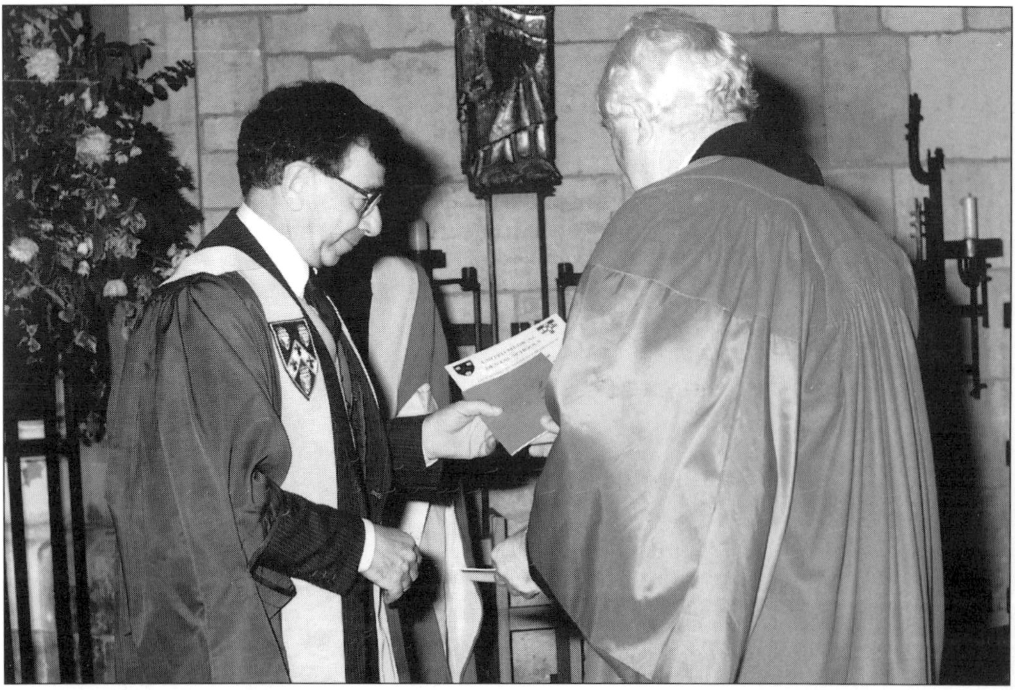

Receiving the Fellowship of the United Medical and Dental Schools in Southwark Cathedral in 1994

dogs using the orthotopic operation – that is, putting the new heart in the normal anatomical place, after first removing the animal's own heart. Shumway was starting to use the drugs that I had investigated in kidney transplantation – 6MP and azathioprine – and was having success with heart transplants.

In Seattle, I saw the work of Belding Scribner, who had developed a method of using an artificial kidney repeatedly so as to keep a patient with irreversible kidney failure alive. Up to that time, the artificial kidney had only been a successful treatment for acute temporary renal failure, from which a patient recovers spontaneously if he can be kept alive for two to four weeks. The limiting factor was the sufferer's blood vessels. For dialysis to work, needles or tubes must be inserted into a suitable artery and vein; but not only are these in short supply, they also become damaged or thrombosed during the process of dialysis itself.

So Scribner and his colleagues had invented a plastic U-tube joining an artery in the forearm to a vein. This could be clamped, uncoupled and joined to the artificial kidney machine for a three- or four-hour treatment, and then joined up again as a shunt between the artery and vein. Eventually this external plastic shunt was superseded by a surgically constructed internal shunt that causes veins in the arm or leg to enlarge so that needles can be easily introduced into them. Such shunts can last for years rather than weeks, as in the early days before Scribner's invention.

A Surgical Possibility

When Patsy, the children and I got back to Boston, the whole of the Brigham transplant group was in agreement that chemical immunosuppression using azathioprine should be moved from the laboratory to the clinic. I was sorry that I had to return to England, my scholarship having run its course, just when clinical applications of my work were to be developed at the Brigham. I was, of course, sad to miss it, but I kept in close contact with Murray and Moore.

Murray's work was eventually given due recognition. After

being out of clinical kidney transplantation for more than twenty years he was awarded the Nobel Prize, together with Donald Thomas, the bone marrow transplanter. There can be no doubt that Murray's work in successful kidney transplantation between identical twins was an extraordinary advance, showing that such surgery could achieve a perfect result, with long-lasting normal function of the kidney. Murray's persistent and meticulous development of this operation paved the way for experiments in immunosuppression in kidney transplantation.

However, after I returned to Britain and azathioprine was being used in clinical transplantation at the Brigham, the early results failed to follow a smooth course. The drug had to be given in doses that were often toxic, and even the rejection of the organ was seldom completely overcome. In 1961 William Goodwin, working in Los Angeles, performed a transplant on a young girl using cyclophosphamide, an anti-cancer drug, as the main immunosuppressant. The patient developed a severe rejection crisis and her kidney became enlarged and stopped functioning. Then Goodwin gave her a short course of large doses of cortisone, which resulted in a dramatic improvement in her condition.

The Brigham group knew of Goodwin's case and added cortisone to the azathioprine chemical immunosuppressant. Clinical renal transplantation then became a reasonable therapeutic option for patients. Thomas Starzl's systematic use of steroids with azathioprine, in a large series of carefully documented cases in the early 1960s, was another important advance in making kidney transplantation an acceptable form of treatment.

This period was an exciting phase in the science of transplantation, and as with most disciplines it was the interaction of the ideas, experiments and observations of a number of people that made it all possible. Murray's identical twin transplants had shown that the procedure was surgically possible. However, the experimental development of immunosuppression was less smooth, and is still not perfect.

Chapter Six
Other People's Organs

We returned to Britain in a small French boat, the *Flandre.* The Atlantic was in continuous storm mode, and my younger daughter Sarah and I seemed to be the only two passengers on board who were not sick, and could still eat. Sadly, we were not able to do justice to the bottles of red and white wine which were always on the table – Sarah was then only two.

Re-entry into Britain was hardly the crash landing I'd been warned it would be. Far from losing my place on the career ladder, I had been offered a number of senior registrar academic posts by visiting British professors while still at the Brigham, not to mention other offers from American professors during my travels.

My Early Attempts

Bill Irvine, professor of surgery at St Mary's Hospital in London, asked me to join the staff there. St Mary's seemed an attractive option, since it already had a programme of kidney transplantation, run by two medical and pathology kidney specialists of international renown, Stanley Peart and my old friend Ken Porter, with whom I had first discussed chemical immunosuppression during my time at the Royal Free Hospital and Buckston Browne Farm.

When I started at St Mary's Hospital, I was eager to get to work on chemical immunosuppression in clinical kidney transplantation. In 1961, some twenty patients had received kidney transplants at St Mary's. They had been treated with x-rays and not one of them had survived. Nevertheless, there was considerable opposition from some of my surgical colleagues to changing the protocol. This seemed extraordinary to me: didn't a 100 per cent mortality rate suggest that our treatment of the patients was not entirely optimal? I suggested that we try azathioprine and cortisone. Fortunately, Peart agreed, and with the help of Porter we were able to start kidney grafting using chemical immunosuppression.

After eighteen months at St Mary's I was offered, and accepted, a senior post as lecturer consultant at Westminster Hospital with my old friend and teacher Harold Ellis, who encouraged me to start a kidney transplant programme there. This proved to be a difficult task. The professor of medicine, Malcolm Milne, was ambivalent and certainly not encouraging but his senior lecturer, Lavinia Loughridge, was anxious to participate and help me with the medical care of patients in kidney failure.

We went ahead and established the ground rules. We did not feel, for instance, that there was enough knowledge or good results to use living related donors. And we knew that kidneys had to be removed from the dead as quickly as possible after the heart had stopped beating, otherwise the organs would be useless. But here we hit a serious snag: the nurse superintendent of the operating theatres would not permit dead bodies to be brought into her operating rooms. So we had to remove the kidneys in the open wards.

Looking back on the procedure, it must have resembled a horror film. Other patients in these large wards would see a team of surgeons rush in, go behind a curtain where a patient had died, and operate on the corpse in an ordinary hospital bed. This was very difficult and blood would often trickle onto the floor, where the patients would see it and be further terrified and upset. The outrage engendered by these goings-on finally made the theatre superintendent give way, and from then on we were able to remove kidneys from cadavers under surgical conditions in an operating theatre, but not without a great deal of resentment from some of the theatre staff.

Since time was always at such a premium in these cases, we occasionally had to remove kidneys from patients who had died in the emergency casualty department. We even turned an ambulance into an operating theatre, when victims of road traffic accidents had died before the ambulance arrived and time was running out. These experiences of operating under terrible conditions made a deep impression on all of us, and helped increase our determination to achieve better working methods.

The early results of kidney transplantation at Westminster were markedly unsuccessful. The kidneys were often too damaged before they were removed and never functioned, and patients were usually too ill when they were accepted for transplantation. But there were a few long-term successes, and these people showed us that it was possible to obtain good results even using kidneys removed from patients where the heart had already stopped beating and the circulation had ceased. But this was obviously not the best way of developing kidney transplantation.

The difficulties surrounding kidney transplantation were a reflection of how precarious and chancy transplantation *per se* had always been. From the beginning of the modern era of transplantation, there have been worries and practical difficulties concerning the source, removal and preservation of organs for transplantation. Structural scaffold-like grafts or prostheses, such as arteries and bones, can be dead or made of inorganic materials such as plastic. But, to be of any use, functioning organs must consist of living cells placed in their normal anatomical relationships to each other.

When David Hume performed the first successful attempts at kidney transplantation in humans at the Brigham in thc early 1950s, he had removed kidneys from patients who had recently died, or used kidneys removed for other reasons. For example, there was an operation popular during the 1950s for treating people with hydrocephalus. This entailed draining the high-pressure fluid that surrounded the brain (and caused the grotesque swelling of the head) via the ureter, the drainage tube of the kidney. The kidney was removed in this procedure; such kidneys were called 'free', and Hume transplanted some of them. The quality of the organs, from the point of view of their ability to function in the recipient, was variable; and undoubtedly some of the kidneys were damaged, despite having been cooled by immersion in ice-cold saline fluid.

There were other, equally fraught ways of obtaining kidneys. In France at about this time the guillotine was still used as a means of execution. René Kuss described how some patients had kidneys transplanted from victims of the guillotine, the criminals having, just prior to execution, given permission for the removal of their kidneys. The whole question of removal of organs from executed prisoners – still a common practice in China and some other countries – has recently been considered by the International Transplantation Society. The current consensus of the international community of transplanters is that the pressures upon criminals due for execution are so intense and dreadful that, even if they have expressed a desire to be donors, organ removal is not considered ethical. It would mean doctors playing a part in the execution, albeit an indirect one. And in some states the death penalty is used for criminal acts which would be regarded as relatively minor in Western countries.

As far as my own kidney transplantation programme at Westminster Hospital was concerned, my wish to make clinical use of the chemical immunosuppression I had developed in the laboratory affected my choice of donors. Since the results were poor, I was only prepared to use kidneys from people who had died, usually from road traffic accidents or major brain haemorrhages, and it was necessary to wait until the heartbeat had stopped before starting to remove the kidneys – the criteria of establishing brain-stem death had not then been clarified. After death the kidney can only remain alive an hour at most without a blood supply, after which it becomes useless for transplantation. And removing kidneys from cadavers, having obtained consent from the next of kin, was an extremely stressful and unsatisfactory procedure. Yet obtaining organs was bound to be an emotive business and we had to steel ourselves to the task.

A Close Encounter

I was now planning a new venture to launch a kidney transplant unit, and chose as its base the Gordon Hospital affiliated to Westminster where I had most of my beds. At this time, in 1963, the transplant world was electrified by the news that kidneys had been transplanted from chimpanzees and baboons to human patients in the United States, and some of these organs had worked well for short periods. The leader of the American programme was Keith Reemtsma in New Orleans, shortly followed by Thomas Starzl in Denver.

I was eager to see this development for myself, and managed to rustle up funds to go to the United States. In New Orleans, in an operation performed by Reemtsma, a young woman received a kidney transplant from a chimpanzee. The transplant was still functioning eight months later, although most of the kidneys from animals had functioned for much shorter periods. The results were worse with baboon kidneys than with those from chimpanzees – hardly surprising, given that chimpanzees are very close to humans in biological terms.

It was inevitable that this odd venture would peter out. None of the baboon kidneys worked for long, and in any case chimpanzees were an endangered species. Nor had the scientific background been developed enough for clinical application. Once back in Britain, however, I was still waxing enthusiastic, and set up a visit to Oliver Graham-Jones, senior vet at London Zoo. He was very anxious to help, and we looked at the feasibility of transplanting a kidney from a baboon to a patient. Special precautions would, of course, be needed, and one of the rooms at the Gordon Hospital was converted so that a baboon could be anaesthetised in it.

The procedure of removing a kidney from a baboon would need to be done under full sterile conditions, and for an adult patient a large baboon would be required. A dummy run was planned, and a huge, immensely strong Dogura baboon with fierce teeth was anaesthetised in the veterinary department of London Zoo, brought to the Gordon Hospital and carried on a stretcher to the special room. The baboon then woke up and we panicked, but Oliver Graham-Jones, with great courage, approached this alarming creature and gave it another shot of anaesthetic. It became tranquil again and was transported rapidly back to the Zoo, where it awoke in due course none the worse for its experience. We soon realised that the time was not ripe for transplants from animals to humans.

Opening Pandora's Box

When I first became interested in transplantation biology in 1959 it never crossed my mind that advances in this area would lead to extraordinary developments in clinical surgery in such a short time, opening up a Pandora's box of difficult, conflicting and sometimes horrific ethical dilemmas. Unfortunately, for there to be any advances in medicine, experiments on animals are necessary, since it is unacceptable to try new and unproven forms of treatment on human patients. Virtually every drug treatment and surgical operation that is carried out in a modern hospital has only become possible through animal experiments. All open-heart surgery, for example, depends on work that has been done in the surgical laboratory. And all the developments in transplantation, both technical and immunological, likewise have only occurred because of serious and responsible experiments on animals. Even insulin, which preserves the lives of diabetics, would not be available without animal experiments.

Animals should only be used in medical research when important information is required to decide if a new treatment should be developed to help sick people. In Britain the regulations governing experiments on animals are so strictly enforced that some able young men and women are deterred by them from entering the fields of academic medicine and surgery. This will ultimately impede progress in alleviating human suffering.

The other main ethical worries, which we have touched on before, concern donors and recipients. To remove organs from a dead person can do them no harm but to remove organs that themselves are dead would be of no value to the recipient. This is the practical dilemma. The tissues of the body are kept alive by blood circulating at 37°C. When the circulation ceases the tissues die. Some are more sensitive than others; the brain is the most vulnerable organ and will not survive more than a few minutes without circulation.

This is the reason why catastrophes occur, for example, as the result of incorrect connection of anaesthetic gas tubes which can suddenly reduce the amount of oxygen carried in the blood. This can, in a few minutes, lead to brain damage that may be permanent, although the other organs may recover, possibly condemning the unlucky survivor of such a disaster to institutional care for the rest of his life (which could be of a normal length).

The trouble is that, with our limited knowledge, doctors and nurses are trained to carry out instant and somewhat violent resuscitation of a patient who has suffered sudden collapse of the circulation. This is graphically depicted in popular television programmes almost nightly. If this resuscitation is successful *before* the brain is damaged, all is well. If the heartbeat cannot be restored then the patient is dead. But there is a limbo state between the two, consisting of a spectrum of brain damage ranging from relatively mild intellectual impairment to severe disability where the individual is incapable of having an independent existence and requires constant care. With more severe brain damage, called a 'vegetative state', the patient is unable to have meaningful contact with other humans, but artificial aids are not necessary to keep the lungs ventilated.

If the brain-stem (where the brain extends from the base of the skull towards the spinal cord in the neck) is destroyed, after attempts at resuscitation and tests show that the damage is irreversible, then the mechanical ventilation of the lungs should be stopped, whether or not organ removal is being considered. Under these circumstances, who can or should be able to give permission for organ removal?

In Britain, if the individual has expressed a clear wish during his or her lifetime that organs should be removed after death to help other individuals, then this is the paramount factor in law and it should not be possible for relatives to reverse it (though, in reality, doctors would not remove organs against the wishes of relatives who were strongly opposed to it). If, however, the individual's wishes are not known, then the next of kin must be approached and their wishes respected. 'The next of kin' are not defined and this term is not restricted to one person; it could be a whole family and one objector could, and has, prevented organ removal, even when the closest relative and the majority were in favour. If there are no next of kin, then the person or institution responsible for the care of the body has authority to say whether or not organs can be removed for transplantation. This would usually be the chief executive of the hospital. Along with all these complexities, if the cause of death is not known, or there may be criminal proceedings, then the coroner has jurisdiction over the body and can order an autopsy. The coroner can also authorise or refuse permission for organs to be removed for transplantation.

In Austria, more than 200 years ago, the Empress Maria Theresa sanctioned a law that anyone dying in hospital was subject to organ removal if the hospital so wished. (This was presumably for the purpose of establishing a diagnosis and studying pathology.) Until recently this law was still in force in Austria, but clearer laws related to transplantation have since been drafted and passed in some countries, and certain states in the US.

Presumed permission to remove organs after death facilitates organ donation. In this so-called 'opting out' system, individuals can register as objectors to organ donation on their own behalf and that of their children, or the relatives can state this when the patient comes into hospital. Otherwise it is legal to remove organs after death without asking further permission. In practice, most of the potential donors are brain-stem dead and on mechanical ventilation, the relatives are usually there, and the question of organ donation can be discussed with them. However, even if there is a law of presumed consent, it would be contrary to medical ethical practice to remove organs from a dead patient if the relatives clearly objected. The law of presumed consent makes it easier to discuss the matter with the relatives; it also becomes more difficult for doctors to evade the complexities of organ donation by using the excuse that it would be inappropriate to ask the relatives.

It requires a sympathetic, experienced individual to discuss the issues of organ donation, brain death and the procedure of organ removal with relatives of patients who have had a sudden catastrophic brain haemorrhage or head injury. But relatives are often pleased that some good can come out of their own dreadful tragedy and that others may be helped. In countries such as Britain, where there is no law of presumed consent, approximately 30 per cent of the population refuses to donate their own organs or those of their relatives. This is a surprisingly high percentage, in view of the widely publicised successes obtained through organ transplantation and the fact that most medical professionals are known to be both ethical and caring. However, those who object to organ donation often seem to change their attitude if they or their loved ones need an organ transplant.

In some countries people refuse permission for organ donation because they do not trust the doctors, and fear that they will not look after the sick individual to the best of their ability if they see them as a potential source of donor organs. In developing countries there is a widespread belief that the body should not be interfered with after death, and that it needs to be intact in order to be reconstituted in heaven. This belief in the sanctity of the body is important and needs to be respected. But, again, those who feel this way will often go to the utmost lengths to obtain an organ for a member of their own family when a transplant is their only chance of survival. Even so, in most Western countries the state has a right to a full post-mortem examination of individuals where the cause of death is not clearly apparent. (In such an examination all the organs are removed, so the body is interfered with anyway.) There is no possibility of avoiding a post-mortem in these circumstances but of course this ruling has nothing to do with organ donation.

Other matters have had to be considered in recent years. For example, is it justifiable to resuscitate the heart and lungs in a patient who is likely soon to become brain dead, where the resuscitation has no purpose other than to keep the organs in a satisfactory condition for transplantation? This has been the subject of much heated discussion in the medical profession and also in the media. The procedure is called 'elective ventilation' and it is carried out only when it has been fully explained to the next of kin and they have given permission. The Department of Health legal advisers in the UK have, however, expressed a view that it may be illegal to resuscitate an individual in order to keep the organs in good condition for transplantation to someone else and so 'elective ventilation' is not now practised in Britain.

The question of money has also entered the debate. Should the donor hospital and its staff be remunerated for the extra work involved in organ removal, the cost of intensive care beds and the stress? A modest remuneration, which goes to the institution not the individuals involved, has now been approved in the UK. Interestingly, Spain has the most successful co-ordination of organ donation in the world, with the highest percentage of donors per million population. The Spanish co-ordinators are well paid, highly motivated, medically qualified individuals, and their sophisticated system of remuneration may well be a factor in their enthusiasm for educating the public and the medical and nursing professions to think of organ donation in patients with brain-stem death.

Defining Death

The Western world changed the practice of organ donation radically, following a CIBA Foundation meeting in London in 1966. The subject was 'organ transplantation' and the existing unsatisfactory state of cadaver organ removal was discussed. Dr Guy Alexandre, from Louvain in Belgium, outlined the criteria of brain death used in Belgium for the condition described in that country as *coma dépassé* (or unconsciousness from which there could be no return). This was, and continues to be, a difficult and emotive subject. No wonder there is often confusion when the media tries to grapple with the complexities of defining death, although non-medical people sometimes seem to have an instinctive grasp of the principles and moral issues involved.

The debate about where the soul lies depends on theological arguments. But, from the point of view of physiology and anatomy, all processes of thought, consciousness and cognitive activity reside in the brain and especially in the higher areas of the brain, the cerebral hemispheres. Nervous impulses conveying signals to and instructions from the brain are essential for the workings of the central nervous system and the organism in general. If the brain is disconnected from the rest of the body by severing the junction between the brain and the spinal cord, at the brain-stem, then the individual is dead. Thus, for example, most people would regard decapitation by the guillotine as evidence of death. A body without a head cannot function; neither can a head without a body. Likewise, execution by hanging breaks the spine at its junction with the skull, and also disconnects the head from the body.

Nerves from the brain-stem are involved in the vital senses of the head – sight, hearing, taste and smell. In establishing brain death, the neurologist therefore needs to be sure that all these pathways have been permanently destroyed. Before there is any consideration of organ donation, the clinical criteria for brain death have to be fulfilled. These are often supplemented by special investigations, such as CT and MR scanning, electrical testing of brain activity, and x-rays of the blood vessels of the brain. We now have accurate imaging techniques which give a clear picture of the actual anatomical state of the brain.

A number of important international conferences have taken place at which neurologists and neurosurgeons have described the criteria necessary to establish permanent destruction of the brain-stem. The tests are, for the most part, clinical, depending on careful observation and eliciting of physical signs. First, the patient must be incapable of spontaneous respiration when the mechanical ventilator is disconnected. Secondly, the presence of any drugs that might produce temporary failure of brain function have to be excluded by testing and the patient's history. Finally, the patient's temperature must be taken, to make sure that cooling of the body has not interfered with brain function. These tests must be performed by two doctors experienced in neurology, who are not part of the transplant team. Having satisfied themselves and recorded the results, they must return after an unspecified interval (usually several hours) to repeat the tests. If there is any doubt about any single test, the patient is not declared brain dead and the doctors wait, perhaps repeating the tests later on.

There has never been a case where brain death has been recorded in this manner and a patient has recovered. In Japan, where the criteria of brain death have only just been accepted in law, many thousands of cases of brain death have been recorded and there has never been a recovery, even after prolonged ventilation. Nevertheless it is hard for doctors and lay people to dissociate themselves completely from the emotions triggered by seeing an individual, often young and without any obvious external injuries, lying as if asleep but with his or her lungs being ventilated mechanically through a tube. It is very difficult to overcome one's initial hope that perhaps this is merely a prolonged sleep from which the patient might miraculously wake.

I still experience these feelings when removing organs from a brain-stem dead individual. Traditionally, death has been diagnosed when the heartbeat and breathing stop, or when a suitably qualified doctor says that the patient is dead. However, with modern surgical advances, it is possible for the heart to be stopped and indeed removed, and the patient kept alive by a heart-lung machine. So, in exceptional circumstances, during open-heart surgery, when providing temporary life support with a heart-lung machine, the traditional criteria for diagnosing death handed down since the time of the ancient Greeks no longer hold.

There is now a remarkable consensus among medical experts in Western countries that brain-stem death is synonymous with the traditional diagnosis of death. And the understanding of this concept of brain-stem death has resulted in improved care of patients with head injuries and brain haemorrhages. In one memorable case in our own practice we had a call from a helpful anaesthetist at a small peripheral hospital where there was a patient with severe brain damage from a motorcycle accident; he was planning to turn the ventilator off and did we want to use the kidneys, since permission had been given? One of my junior surgical colleagues enquired into the details, politely pointed out that the criteria of brain death had not been satisfied, and suggested that the youngster was sent to Addenbrooke's Hospital for a neurological assessment. The doctors in the small hospital were surprised but complied with this suggestion. The cause of the brain damage was found to be a haemorrhage under the lining of the skull. When this was removed by the neurosurgeons the patient rapidly recovered and walked out of hospital! This was an excellent illustration of how important it is to fulfil all the criteria of brain death before contemplating turning off the ventilator, and was an unusual success resulting from the needs of transplantation.

However, once it has been ascertained that the brain is irreversibly destroyed and the patient is dead, is it justifiable to remove the organs while the circulation is intact and the ventilator is still working? Or should the ventilator first be disconnected, and the heartbeat have stopped? At first the debate went back and forth on this, but then it was pointed out that waiting until the heart stopped would mean that all the organs that might be transplanted would be severely damaged because they would not have a proper oxygenated blood supply. In fact, the heart would not be suitable for transplantation under these circumstances, while the liver would be damaged badly and the kidneys moderately.

The practice was therefore established of explaining to the relatives that death had occurred but requesting that the ventilator should continue to be used until the organs were removed so that they would be of use to potential recipients. This has been the pattern in most Western countries, including Canada and the US, since the late 1960s. Whenever the criteria of brain death have been challenged, they have stood fast as an absolute and reliable instrument for clinical diagnosis. In an infamous *Panorama* programme put out by the BBC in the early 1980s, four cases of brain damage were presented from America, all of whom recovered, but in none of them had the criteria of brain death been established correctly. This programme created great confusion in the minds of the public and a catastrophic fall in organ donation, which took many months to recover.

Traditional laws do not cater for brain death and organ donation, except in a rather general sense. For example, English common law maintains that a dead body has no property but is in the custody of the relatives or whoever is designated locally (such as a hospital superintendent). A body cannot be bought or sold. The question of whether or not to remove organs from a body should depend entirely on the wishes of the deceased in his or her lifetime. But often those wishes are not known; it is only recently that they have sometimes been recorded on a donor card or a computer. As we have seen, defining death as simply a cessation of life's processes is unhelpful; the criteria of brain-stem death have therefore helped to focus ideas on this subject.

The laws governing organ donation from a living donor have also, in general, been ill defined. According to traditional Hippocratic teaching, a doctor is obliged not to do any harm: removing an organ from a healthy person is clearly a harmful and potentially dangerous procedure. But, as has been explained in the case of identical twins, failure to help a dying relative could also be regarded as causing deep psychological harm. So where should we draw the line on organ donation? Whereas removal of one healthy kidney may be an acceptable risk, what are the ethics of removing half a liver, or a lobe of lung, which are more dangerous operations? These are all questions which have been raised, as has the idea of deliberately conceiving a baby in the hope that it will prove to be a suitable bone marrow donor for a sibling afflicted by leukaemia.

The Gift of Life

For a parent to give a kidney to a child suffering from kidney disease would seem reasonable. There is a sacrifice involved, the operation is not without danger, it is painful and the results are not perfect, but, having understood all these things, many parents will elect to give a kidney. However, one father recently asked to give his second kidney to his second child, thereby sacrificing all his kidney tissue. He planned to survive, presumably on dialysis, or a kidney graft, but no British transplant surgeon would take up his offer.

In July 1996 a German transplant surgeon in Lübeck, Professor Jochem Hoyer, gave a kidney to a twenty-nine-year-old man whose identity he did not know, in order to demonstrate the value of live organ donation, which accounts for only 5 per cent of all transplantations a year. Professor Hoyer said he had donated his kidney to give moral support to all those who have to decide whether or not to help a related person who needs a kidney.

What relationship is needed between donor and recipient for a doctor to be prepared to proceed with live organ donation? Husband-to-wife and wife-to-husband kidney donation has become popular in the United States, and is now being practised in other Western countries. But can the transplant team be sure that no moral or financial pressure has been exerted on the family member donor to give a kidney?

In some countries the recipient is only offered a kidney from a cadaver if there is no suitable living donor. But is it reasonable to put pressure on somebody who is perfectly healthy to donate an organ? There is sometimes little love lost between siblings in a family, and even between parents and children there are occasions when there is scant evidence of love.

Having considered these matters, how do we feel about payment for organs? This is generally regarded as unethical. However, in a developing country the payment for a kidney could transform the life of a poor peasant on the verge of starvation so that his whole family could have a better standard of living and he could perhaps give his children an education. Should he not be permitted to sell his kidney, just as he would sell something he had made? The argument against this is that commerce in organs demeans the whole process of transplantation and there is a likelihood of middlemen or organ brokers cheating the donor and the recipient for personal gain. For these reasons, the government of India recently outlawed this procedure. This was an important step since in India, while many thousands of organ transplants were carried out in which the donor was paid and the recipient was rich, there were not many instances of organ donation from rich to poor.

However, it is still legal in India to accept an organ from a non-blood-relative spouse and there are cases of marriages of convenience where the dowry may pay not only for the spouse but also for a kidney. It is difficult to control this practice of marrying to circumvent the law on paying for organs. And the complexities of the divorce settlement, when marriages break down, will no doubt occupy a great many lawyers.

These considerations are worrying enough, but for somebody dying of malfunction of a vital organ a healthy replacement organ is valuable beyond price. There is therefore a temptation in some evil people to obtain organs by means of coercion or of murder. Of course, this would not happen unless there was complicity on the part of doctors and nurses and unless the institutions involved were shielded from public scrutiny. In Eastern Europe, Latin America, China, the Middle East and South-East Asia there have been many reports of people being abducted and having a kidney removed; or having a kidney removed together with an appendix when the kidney was perfectly normal; or worse, people being kidnapped or murdered and their organs removed. It has been very difficult to authenticate any of these allegations. If such criminal practices occur, the perpetrators must cover their tracks very cleverly and bribe or terrorise all those in the know so that they keep their mouths shut.

We need very strict safeguards against such dreadful criminal acts. I suggested compulsory registration many years ago and this has now been taken up in Britain. Details of the donor operation, what was wrong with the donor, who the surgeons were, where the organ went, who the recipient was, and which institution did the recipient operation all have to be registered in Britain. The donor and recipient registration forms are legal documents, like birth and death certificates; and this has been reassuring for the public and also for doctors involved in organ transplantation.

An extraordinary heart transplant took place in Michigan, USA, in September 1994. Chester Szuber, a fifty-eight-year-old man with severe heart disease was listed for a heart graft. Some months later there was a dreadful tragedy in his family when his twenty-two-year-old daughter Patti was involved in a road traffic accident in which her brain was destroyed and she was therefore put on a ventilator. A donor card was found in her handbag. Chester and Patti's doctors conferred and it was clear to them all that Patti had declared her wish to be an organ donor and that in the circumstances she would have wanted her father to be the recipient. The operation took place and was a success. Since then, Chester has campaigned with great vigour, persistence and a special emotional strength engendered by the pain of losing a daughter and the ultimate gift she gave him.

As for the problem of organ donation, I suppose the only way of improving the situation is by further educating the public. And I do believe that an opting-out law would make the whole question of organ donation easier for the relatives and the doctors and nurses involved. Sometimes ingenious promotional devices are required, to bring the subject of organ donation to the forefront of people's minds. For example, in order to help publicise donor cards, a Cambridge milliner called Geraldine, who was also a model, once produced a wonderful hat made from about 350 donor cards. She accompanied me to Royal Ascot, wearing the hat.

Quality of Life

When organ transplantation was in its infancy, the perception in the minds of the medical profession and the public was of an unnatural and hazardous endeavour resulting in much publicity but conferring little benefit to the patients. The many failures encouraged this view and the successes were ignored, except by those involved in the care of the patients.

A relative who has donated a kidney has made a deliberate, altruistic choice and although aware of the possibility of failure, expects success rather in the same way as the soldier going into battle or a football team going into the World Cup Final. A happy outcome is usually a continuing joy for the donor but if the graft is rejected there is disappointment and a feeling of being let down. When unrelated donors in prison 'volunteered' to give a kidney, some felt that this was repaying a debt to the community, but there were also stories of prisoner donors, after release, knocking on the doors of the recipients of their kidneys demanding financial compensation. This was one of the reasons why the use of kidneys from prisoners was stopped.

When an organ is removed from a dead donor, the relatives will often worry and hope for a good outcome in the transplant operation. Usually identification of the recipient for the donor family is avoided because contact can lead to a variety of tensions and disputes and once again, there is the possibility of the donor family requesting financial compensation, although this is unlikely. The recipient also has feelings of sadness and guilt and of gratitude if the donor was dead and sense of love and continuing thanks to a living donor for this supreme gift.

Since organ transplantation was such a strange and special form of treatment, after a successful operation the patients were regarded by many as unemployable and were refused their old jobs. The patients also felt sometimes that they would be chronic invalids. This is not true and many patients have been restored to full and extremely active life. Often the organ graft is considered as a second chance and many patients live life in a fuller sense, both physically and emotionally, than before the operation. In order to encourage this self respect and show the community that full rehabilitation after an organ graft was possible, my colleague and friend, Maurice (Taffy) Slapak, when he became director of kidney transplantation in Portsmouth, inaugurated the Transplant Olympics. This was a wonderful concept which has flourished since 1978 when the first Games were held. Patients compete in a wide variety of athletic events, there are social reunions, and the idea has spread rapidly so that now fifty countries have their own national Transplant Games and every two years an international Olympics is held in a different country. This has been one of the most important contributions to the morale of transplant patients. The publicity attending these Games, where the athletic performances are often outstandingly good, has convinced many members of the public who previously were uncertain to become donors; it has given the patients and potential patients a feeling of optimism, and hopefully will convince employers that a transplant patient with a well functioning graft can hold down a job and often work as well or better than before he or she became ill. Taffy Slapak, a distinguished sportsman himself, has worked enthusiastically over many years to develop the Transplant Olympics and he can be proud of the result.

Chapter Seven
The Cambridge Connection

In 1964 as a lecturer, and second-in-command to Harold Ellis in the University Department of Surgery at the Gordon Hospital, I began to feel that it was essential to have my own department to develop transplantation both experimentally and clinically, and I applied for a variety of chairs of surgery. I was shortlisted for the Chair at St Vincent's Hospital in Melbourne, and members of the faculty came over to England to watch me at work and determine whether I could operate – and, more subtly, to ensure that I did not have politically disturbing tendencies. (They seemed to think that all English academics were Communists.) Having satisfied themselves as to my surgical competence and moderate political views, they offered me the Chair.

In the meantime, I had applied for the Chair of Surgery in Cambridge. This was a new post, although at the turn of the century two surgeons at Addenbrooke's Hospital, Cambridge, had been given the honorary title of professor. They did not have departments in the modern sense and the post had not been renewed. In 1960 Cambridge defied the British Medical Association on conditions of service, and were not prepared to pay professors the normal salary. The BMA had therefore blacklisted them and advertisements for Cambridge posts appeared surrounded by a black border, to put would-be applicants off this 'cheap-jack' Chair.

I was not, however, in a position to choose, and so was pleased when I was asked to look around. I wanted to stay in England for family as well as professional reasons, so I asked the Melbourne University authorities if they would mind waiting until I heard the outcome of the Cambridge post. This request did not please them, but there was nothing to be done about that. In the event, there was no interview for the Cambridge job, but one evening when my wife and I were at the local cinema, the Vice-Chancellor of Cambridge University phoned our house and spoke to our Danish au pair girl, asking if I would mind being available on the telephone next morning. My wife asked if he had said anything else, and the au pair said she thought it was something to do with a job.

The next morning, the vice-chancellor informed me that the electors to the Chair would like me to come to Cambridge, beginning in the academic year of 1965. I accepted. I was sorry to leave London, where I had worked most of my life, but Cambridge had wonderful departments of basic science, and I thought there would be the possibility of developing transplantation there, although in the 1960s Addenbrooke's was little more than a glorified cottage hospital, with a small postgraduate school and aspirations for a clinical school.

So, in October 1965 we moved to Cambridge, although I had no department to move into. I had, however, general surgical facilities offered to me and an office on top of a terraced house near the hospital. In the lower part of this house lived an Indian family, so my office was permanently infused with strong curry odours that sometimes took away my usual hearty appetite for curry. I managed to get a typewriter for my secretary, who came up with me from Westminster. And that was it!

The prospect of renal transplantation was greeted with indifference or hostility by most of my new colleagues, but supported by a few. In any case, the programme soon got underway. David Evans, a young kidney specialist, joined me in the department of surgery – an act of 'professional suicide', according to his colleagues. However, thanks to his superb efforts, dialysis and the care of patients reached a high standard.

We developed close contact with Peter Medawar's department and had regular meetings, either in Cambridge or at Northwick

Park Hospital, on the outskirts of London. Valerie Joysey set up the tissue typing laboratory in Cambridge and was a constant source of enthusiasm and information.

Tissue typing is of central importance in organ transplantation. First of all the red cell groups must be compatible and it is essential that the patient does not have antibodies against the donor white blood cells. This can happen after multiple pregnancies, blood transfusion or previous transplants. The nearer the match of the white blood cell types, the better the result of the transplant. Normally parent-to-child will always be at least half-matched; and sibling-to-sibling will have a one in four chance of a perfect match, a one in four chance of no match, and a one in two chance of a half-match.

Two Memorable Patients

So I settled in. In 1966 a patient called John Neil was sent to me by my friend and colleague in Belfast, Dr Molly McGewan. He had end-stage kidney disease, a complication of which had left him completely blind. Having received a new kidney, his progress was satisfactory from the start. He went back to Belfast where, despite his blindness, he was able to enjoy a very full life. Every time I visited Northern Ireland I would meet him and his family. He had an extraordinary serenity of spirit and even when the Troubles were at their worst in Belfast he still managed to retain a cheerful and hopeful outlook. He eventually died of a heart attack, thirty-two years after his kidney operation, having been a beacon of encouragement to us that transplantation could provide a wonderful cure when all went well.

I met another one of my more memorable transplant patients in 1966, just before tissue typing became available. At this time kidney transplantation was still a major procedure, but Nigel McLeod, a tall, handsome soldier, seemed to be up to it. Nigel was a young man when he became ill with Bright's disease of the kidneys. He received his new kidney in Addenbrooke's Hospital on 4 November 1966 from an unrelated road traffic accident victim. Nigel recovered and the kidney was functioning well, when he developed severe pneumonia, which only partially responded to antibiotics: an abscess formed, he became exceedingly ill, and we thought he was going to die. We removed a portion of Nigel's rib overlying the abscess under a local anaesthetic, as he was too sick for a general anaesthetic. The pus was drained with Nigel sitting up since he could not lie down because of his breathlessness.

Nigel recovered very slowly and was left with a hole in his chest that connected to his lungs. Despite this, he became stronger, his kidney functioned well and he finally left hospital. It was then that he discovered his phenomenal party trick: when he inhaled the smoke from a cigarette, closed his mouth and exhaled, the smoke would come out of the hole in his chest. He became very skilled at it, discovering that it caused great interest and amusement among fellow regulars in the pubs. A really impressive jet of smoke shooting out of his chest would be rewarded with a pint of beer.

We offered to close the hole, but he was reluctant to lose these benefits. It was only when all the locals had witnessed the smoke trick several times, and no longer wished to see it repeated, that he came into hospital and had it dealt with by Ben Milstein, my old teacher from Guy's. Since then Nigel has done very well. He married and remained in good health, apart from a skin cancer which had to be removed twenty years after his operation – a grim reminder that, even years after a transplant, patients on low-dose immunosuppression are still at risk from infection and development of growths. He is now our longest surviving organ transplant recipient, still going strong after thirty-two years.

The Young Army Cadet

The year 1966 saw another extraordinary case. On a beautiful July day during an idyllic summer in southern England, a young army cadet called Alistair was involved in an exercise with his company. Having marched and run many miles in the hot sun, they were dismissed for lunch. Alistair and his companions, exhausted and sweating but in good humour, decided to have a pub lunch. They washed the veal and ham pie down with a pint of cider, and then another pint was suggested, and no one was willing to be seen as less macho than the others so a second pint was drunk.

The boys dispersed and Alistair wandered back towards the rest of the company but, since he still had half an hour of lunch-break left, he decided to lie down in the meadow. Sleep hit him between the eyes, a deep, peaceful and happy sleep. A jeep was driving across the meadow and the driver didn't see Alistair in the long grass. The impact of the jeep as it hit him across his abdomen must have been a very rude awakening. The agony in his stomach took his breath away. Alistair had no idea what had happened but the occupants of the jeep had felt the bump and the cadets jumped out, placed him on the seat of the jeep and drove to the nearest hospital. An emergency surgical team was called. The surgeon looked grave. Alistair's body had gone a deathly white, which made his sunburned face look grotesque. His pulse felt like a fluttering thread and his blood pressure was below 90. His abdomen was swollen, with the tyre marks of the jeep across it, and it was getting more and more distended, making him appear pregnant.

An emergency operation was performed and there was so much blood inside the abdominal cavity that it could not be measured; all units of group O blood in the hospital were quickly used up in replacing the shed blood and more was sent for. The cause of this dreadful haemorrhage was a star-like rupture of the liver, which had been squashed by the jeep's tyre against Alistair's spine. The splits were like crevices deep in the right side of the liver and blood was pouring from them. There seemed to be little that could be done so the surgeon inserted a cotton gauze roll into the middle of the hole and packed it around the liver, in front and behind, and the flow of blood lessened. The theatre sister said she had run out of packs but, since this procedure seemed to be stabilising Alistair's condition, the surgeon requested that a clean sheet be brought in and he tore this up and used it as further packing.

Now, to the surprise of the surgeons, nurse and anaesthetists, the blood loss had dropped to a mere ooze, so the surgeon quickly closed the abdomen, reached for the phone and rang Addenbrooke's. I was on duty and agreed to accept the youngster as an emergency case. He was placed in an ambulance and driven gently but speedily to Addenbrooke's. I read the notes and my heart sank. Although alive and conscious, Alistair looked dreadful and I felt we should give him more blood transfusions, but I would have to bite the bullet and remove the packs, as otherwise they would cause a fatal infection. Removing them, however, could well result in a fatal haemorrhage.

Twenty-four hours after the first operation Alistair was brought to the Addenbrooke's operating theatre. By this time news of his arrival had got round the hospital and the other surgeons soon came to watch, curious to see by what means the new Professor of Surgery would cause the death of the fatally injured cadet. Alistair was anaesthetised and wheeled into the theatre. The atmosphere was tense and I was terrified. I removed the sutures from the abdomen and gently started to remove the bits of sheet. Where they were stuck with blood I irrigated the area with warm saline and gently pulled them out, one by one, and then the packs. It was extraordinary but there was no fresh bleeding. Only one pack remained and by this time I could see a huge rent in the middle of the liver. As I pulled the last pack out, it did not come away on its own – stuck to it was the whole of the right half of the liver. The most astounding fact was that there was no bleeding from the remaining surface apart from a few small spots, which were easily dealt with by simple stitches. I put two drains in the abdomen, which I closed, and smiled at my colleagues, who had kindly come to witness a drama that never occurred.

Two weeks later Alistair left hospital with normal liver function and returned to the cadet force. This sixteen-year-old boy with a dreadful liver injury had taught me a number of lessons. Besides the well-known adage, while there is life, there is hope, the chief lesson was the importance of using packs to stop the bleeding, in order to gain vital extra time.

Previous results in cases of liver trauma had been fairly disastrous. The accident victim came into hospital in a similar state to Alistair, and was usually operated on by a surgeon who had little experience of liver injuries because it was not a very common emergency in any one institution. There was seldom sufficient blood available and the anaesthetists were also unfamiliar with this kind of injury. The surgeon would realise that the bleeding was coming from a deep crevice-like split but would be unable to see exactly which blood vessel was leaking. In order to get a view, he would probe the crevice, which made the bleeding worse. The patient usually expired on the operating table. The idea of packing a bleeding wound is an old one; packs were used in war surgery for centuries but had a bad reputation because they led to infection, which usually proved fatal. Now, however, we had antibiotics and if the packing could stop the fatal progression of haemorrhage, the body would be given time to make new clotting factors which had been used up in the first haemorrhage. This technique also allowed time for the critically ill patient to be transferred to a unit where there was experience of liver surgery, with skilled surgeons and anaesthetists and a blood bank that could cope with huge demands.

I instituted this policy for the treatment of liver injuries in Addenbrooke's and patients were sent from long distances, sometimes by air, with their lungs mechanically ventilated. Every patient who was sent survived after removal of the packs; sometimes half the liver needed to be removed but often this was not necessary. I published this method of treatment, which was initially scorned because it was unorthodox and felt to be old fashioned. But antibiotics have changed the way in which patients can be managed and over the years it has become possible to diagnose the extent of liver damage by CT scanning without having to open up the abdomen. Some patients thus survive without an operation who would have died if they had been anaesthetised and subjected to surgery.

Besides the importance of using packs to gain extra time, I learnt once again that because the major surgical literature emanates from North America, most American surgeons don't read European medical reports; the early publications from Addenbrooke's on liver trauma are therefore very seldom cited in later, much larger series reported from America. If medical cases are published in non-English language journals, their chances of being ignored are even greater.

Adventures in Argentina

Shortly after I came to Cambridge I received a letter from an Argentinean friend asking me if I would help him start kidney transplantation in Buenos Aires. He invited me to stay in the Italian hospital there and perform a transplant using a kidney donated by a mother to her daughter. When I arrived in Buenos Aires my accommodation was in the residential part of the hospital, under the care of the nuns who were also nursing sisters. Everything was spotlessly clean and tidy. My clothes were whisked away and washed and ironed to perfection.

In the event, the kidney transplant operation proceeded satisfactorily, although the large number of people in the operating theatre jostling each other to get a view made it difficult to maintain sterility and the background noise did not help concentration. However, all went well, my hosts departed and I went to my quarters. In the early hours of the morning I was woken by a nun who asked me to come quickly to see the patient with the kidney transplant.

When I arrived the nuns were looking worried, the patient was deathly pale and blood was coming from the wound drain. Bleeding after a kidney transplant is a well-known complication and it usually stops when a blood transfusion is given so I requested that we put up some blood. They shook their heads.

I said, 'Why not?'

They said, 'The blood is kept in the fridge.'

I said, 'Well, can we get it?'

They said, 'No. The fridge is locked.'

I said, 'Well, let's unlock it.'

They said, 'No, it's impossible. The Mother Superior has the key and she lives in a different location, in a nunnery some miles out of town.'

I couldn't believe that there was no access to blood in the

middle of the night. But it was true. So we replaced the blood loss with plasma and saline and, although shocked, the patient became a little more stable and her blood pressure rose.

I asked if we could contact the Mother Superior earlier and I was told no, it was impossible. However, she would arrive at about eight a.m.; so, from seven onwards, I was pacing up and down the hospital reception hall waiting for her. At last the Mother Superior came, and I rushed up to her, imploring with one word, 'Sanguina, sanguina.' It took a little time for her to realise that I was not a maniac, after which she hurried to the refrigerator and opened the locked compartment so that we could obtain blood. As soon as the patient received a transfusion she improved and the bleeding stopped. Again I had learnt a lesson – this time on how important it is for the back-up and infrastructure to be appropriate for the operations carried out in an institution. It doesn't matter how well trained the surgeon is: without this back-up, patients will perish.

Skiing and Immunology

Around this time, Professor Walter Brendl, head of the experimental surgical department in Munich, decided to study immunology as a major thrust in his department's work. He therefore organised an immunology meeting in Kitzbühel in the Austrian Alps, to which a number of scientists from different nations were invited, including Medawar.

The first meeting was held in 1968, just after the first human heart transplant had been performed by Christiaan Barnard in Cape Town, South Africa. Organ transplantation was then achieving world-wide publicity and also some opprobrium, due to many subsequent failures of heart transplants. I was fortunate to be invited to the first gathering in Kitzbühel and have been a regular participant in subsequent meetings.

The Munich department had very little experience of transplantation immunology but Walter Brendl was interested in developing anti-lymphocyte serum and made important contributions in producing a better version than had previously been available. He was a charismatic and dedicated person, and worked extremely hard in starting a new department and carrying it forward to become the most prestigious experimental surgical department in Germany. He had been severely injured in the Russian campaign in the Second World War but, with characteristic courage, he had refused to let his wounds hold him back, and he was an enthusiastic and fearless skier. A pattern soon evolved at Kitzbühel – of skiing in the morning (with students from the Munich department teaching novice overseas skiers the rudiments of the sport), followed by several hours of friendly but disciplined discourse on transplantation immunology in the afternoon.

The German students learnt quickly, and soon started teaching some of the visitors immunology. Regrettably, the visitors' prowess at skiing did not match the Germans' swift progress in immunology. The cost of holding the meetings in Kitzbühel became too great and later meetings were held in Axams, near Innsbruck. It was here that I met Raimond Margreiter, the transplant surgeon at Innsbruck teaching hospital. We became friends and every year I stayed a few extra days in his house.

Raimond Margreiter is a prince among men, an outstanding intellect, a surgeon who had transplanted every organ that could be transplanted, and also an expert in bone marrow transplantation. As well as being a superb technical surgeon, he was an extremely thoughtful scientist. In addition to these formidable characteristics, Margreiter was an international standard sportsman for whom no challenge was too great. As a student he was in the national Austrian competitive downhill ski team. He was an expert climber and a member of the Austrian Everest expedition, who scaled the summit for the first time without the help of extra oxygen. He was also a 'white water' canoeist and the first in the world to circumnavigate the upper reaches of the Amazon single-handed.

Needless to say, a man of such distinction and achievement was hero-worshipped by most of his fellow citizens and hated by a few who yapped at his heels like hyenas looking for weak points and being disappointed. Margreiter was a forthright champion of the cause of his patients and the need to develop transplantation in

Austria. After one of the Brendl immunology meetings I was enjoying a short skiing holiday when I was summoned from the ski slopes by Margreiter to join him in carrying out the first liver transplant in Austria.

He had a suitable patient, a forty-year-old woman, waiting as a recipient. A donor had been declared brain dead and permission had been given to remove the liver for transplantation. He asked me to do the operation, with him as first assistant. The set-up in the operating theatre in Innsbruck was excellent, the theatre sister very experienced, and – despite the language difference – we managed without too much difficulty. I was surprised when the lady anaesthetist started preparing the patient by acupuncture needling of the ear. This seemed to put her in a trance and then morphia was given and a general anaesthetic supplemented the acupuncture. I think this must have been the first liver transplant assisted at least partly by acupuncture anaesthesia.

At the end of the procedure the patient's condition was stable and extremely satisfactory and we were pleased to note that the new liver looked beautiful when it was reperfused with blood. I was due to go home the next day. The surgical team was exhausted and the patient was in intensive care so I said goodbye to Margreiter and returned home. The following day he called me with the dreadful news that the woman had suddenly died. Apparently the cause was excessive potassium administration. This was a salutary and tragic warning that, although the surgical team may be exhausted and unable to continue the standard of care required after the operation, there should always be trained people available who are capable of caring for a patient with the same expertise after the operation as during the procedure.

Tolerance through the Liver

After the move to Cambridge, I had no facilities for research but, thanks to the generosity of Dr Richard Keynes, I was allowed to work at the Agricultural Research Station at Babraham, where he was director. There I met Richard Binns, who had just completed his thesis on the production of tolerance in the pig by intra-uterine embryo injection (a direct application of the experiments carried out in the 1950s by Billingham, Brent and Medawar). The behaviour of his tolerant animals when they received donor kidneys seemed highly relevant to my work, and we found that they were less likely to reject kidneys than skin from the same donor.

In the late 1960s we heard of some liver grafting experiments performed in pigs by John Terblanche and Joe Peacock in Bristol and Henri Garnier and J.-P. Clot in Paris. I had yet to do any experimental liver grafting, although Francis Moore had been developing the technique in dogs at the Brigham when I was there. Some of the pigs given liver allografts in the experiments in Bristol and Paris survived for surprisingly long periods. This was of particular interest in view of the work we had done in collaboration with Binns.

So we set about developing the technique of orthotopic (correct anatomical position) liver grafting in pigs, a task that demanded considerable perseverance in the face of many disappointments. Eventually, however, we showed that liver grafts in pigs were rejected less aggressively than any other transplant tissue that had so far been studied, and that a successful liver graft could make the animal tolerant so that they accepted other tissues from the same donor without any drug treatment.

This was, in fact, the first demonstration of operational tolerance in immunologically mature animals without the use of immunosuppressive agents. The concept was confirmed more elegantly by my colleagues Franz Zimmermann, Naoshi Kamada, Hugh Davies and Bruce Roser in liver grafts between different inbred strains of rat with controlled tissue mismatches.

After many generations of in-breeding, rats form a strain with each individual having the same tissue type. It is therefore possible to transplant skin and organs between strains with a knowledge of the tissue type of the individuals. Skin and most organs grafted across a major tissue-type barrier are rejected in seven to ten days. The grafted liver, however, can overcome rejection and we were amazed to find that tolerance occurred.

A Trip Behind the Iron Curtain

Soon after taking up my post in Cambridge, I was approached by the Foreign Secretary of the Royal Society to ask whether I would care to join Sir Peter Medawar and Professor James Gowans on a cultural trip to Russia, to cover the subject of tissue and organ transplantation. Medawar and Gowans were distinguished scientists and I was the junior member. We were to lecture on transplantation biology and clinical organ grafting.

I was delighted to accept, and the three of us flew to Moscow. The Cold War was at its height. We had been warned by the Foreign Office not to get involved in any discussions of a political nature, but in the Soviet Union at that time virtually any conversation could be regarded by the KGB as politically unacceptable. Jim Gowans and I shared a room and Medawar had a separate room. Jim and I noticed a large bowl of flowers in the middle of our huge, freezing Victorian hotel room and we would deliberately address comments to this bowl of flowers on certain things that we found unsatisfactory in the Soviet Union. We were convinced that there was a microphone hidden in the flower bowl. However, we had heard the story of some Western visitors with similar suspicions who had unbolted the stand holding the table (which they thought concealed a microphone). Apparently it turned out that the bolts had been holding a huge chandelier on to the ceiling of the ballroom below, and there was a devastating crash when the glass edifice fell on to the marble floor. We therefore did not try any similar experiments with our flower bowl but remained suspicious nevertheless.

We visited various biological institutes in Moscow and gave lectures. On one of these occasions Medawar gave a brilliant lecture and was cheered by all the students, but then an older man got up and angrily challenged Medawar, stating that his science was all confused because he didn't do the skin grafting properly. This critic was Demikopf, a surgeon who had transplanted extra heads onto dogs (experiments which had earned him notoriety in the West). He was also a follower of the political biology of Trofim Lysenko, derived from the theory of Jean Baptiste de Lamarck that acquired characteristics could be inherited: for example, giraffes acquired long necks in order to reach food high in the treetops. This idea had long been discredited, following the observations and reasoning of Charles Darwin and Alfred Wallace who suggested, rather more logically, that giraffes who happened to have long necks would have been the sole survivors when food could only be found in the tops of trees.

The political control of biological science was a terrible handicap for the Soviet Union, causing a stagnation of innovative experiments and disastrous results in agriculture. Science is an area where political interference usually does harm, although one has to admit that political distribution of funds and designation of research priorities can be extremely helpful. In physics, for example, this political backing allowed the Russians to be the first into space with Sputnik, and the Americans to counter with the first man on the moon.

In Moscow I met the surgeon who had translated my book on kidney transplantation into Russian, where it had been published as a pirate edition. He was very proud of his translation. However, I reminded him of the letters that my English publishers had sent him and he said that I need not worry because all the money would be paid to me before the end of my trip.

We visited Lumumba University, named after the African patriot who opposed Belgian imperialism. Many students from Africa were educated in the Soviet Union, but just before we arrived there had been racist riots against black students by the Russian students, so there was an ominous tension in the air. We were ushered into the university director's office and subjected to the usual long spiel about how wonderful the Russians were to poor deprived peoples. I found it difficult to take this type of propaganda and was drifting into a gentle sleep when Medawar nudged me and told me to wake up and listen to more of 'le mumbo-jumbo'.

We visited the hospital of the first surgical unit where the director was Professor Petrovski, who was also the Minister of Health. He had thick carpets and a refrigerator well stocked with caviar and vodka. No doubt he wrote letters to the Minister of Health, explaining how poor Professor Petrovski at the surgical unit needed various supplies. Wearing his other hat in the Ministry, we imagined these requests would be dealt with in a sympathetic manner: 'Poor Petrovski, we'll send him the caviar and vodka and make sure his carpets are appropriate for his status.' We travelled to Kiev and gave more lectures. The biological sciences were not regarded as a priority and it was only in Moscow that the laboratory and hospital equipment in any way approached those of the West.

Later we flew an enormous distance to Novasobiesk where there was a huge science postgraduate university and institute. The director there seemed to have more freedom than the scientists we had met in the cities, and he welcomed us to his house and showed us round his beautiful garden. Although it was October we were able to bathe in the Obskier, a huge artificial lake created by the damming of the River Ob. The surroundings of Novasobiesk were beautiful, with extensive pine forests similar to Canada. However, we were only allowed to visit certain parts of the institute; presumably there were areas where secret work relating to armaments and weapons was in progress.

For me, as a junior professor of surgery, this trip was a revelation – not only because of what I learnt from the Russians, but also because I was in close contact with two of the most distinguished scientists in transplantation biology. I found their rigorously logical approach, combined with their openness to innovation, fascinating and I have tried to adopt these attitudes in my own work, although in clinical surgery one does not have the same freedom to choose experimental models that are available to a pure scientist.

Jim Gowans had to leave before the end of the trip for family reasons and Peter Medawar left shortly afterwards as he had developed a bad cold. This left me both the most junior and senior member of the commission and I travelled with the lady Intourist guide, a Communist Party member who took her politics very seriously. Together we went to Odessa and stayed in one of the grand old hotels, its decor unchanged since Victorian times – there was even a palm court orchestra playing. It was a very romantic setting but dialectic materialism was the main preoccupation of my Intourist lady. She castigated me for our continued belief in religion in the West. I told her that it was sad but religion seemed to be declining in the West, whereas in the Soviet Union, of course, it was extremely strong. She coloured and replied furiously that there was no such thing as religion in the Soviet Union. I begged to differ and explained that I had seen a picture of her god in every office we had visited; in fact it was usually the same picture. When she realised that I was referring to Lenin she became silent, the hushed and solemn silence of religious observance. 'Oh, Lenin, you mean'. It was interesting that, for the party faithful, Communism seemed to fill the spiritual void in a people who are naturally deeply religious.

Back in Moscow, after a long wait in an office, I was presented with a shopping bag full of roubles in payment for the pirated edition of my book. I could not take the money out so I bought a hat for my wife and two tins of caviar. The rest of the roubles were deposited in the Moscow People's Savings Bank where I suppose they dissolved away. I returned home after six weeks, very relieved to get on a British Airways plane. I had not been able to communicate directly with my wife although there had been indirect messages from mutual friends connected with the British Embassy. It had been an extremely educative experience but I was glad that I did not live in the Soviet Union.

Thomas Starzl – A Giant of Modern Surgery

On my return, I went back to our experiments in liver grafting in pigs where the results were fascinating, but unravelling their significance was proving difficult. Nevertheless the experiments gave us confidence in the liver transplant operation in the pig, where the anatomy is similar to that of humans. All of this experimentation was, of course, the foothills; clinical liver transplantation was our Everest, and Thomas Starzl was the first to scale it, in 1963. The early results were dismal, but this did not put him off. There are not many, if any, figures in the field of contemporary surgery or surgical history who can compare with Starzl. Now in his seventies, his energy is still quite extraordinary, his intellect sharp and swift, his memory for minute details astounding, and he has a laser-like ability to focus his attention on the cutting edge of transplantation biology. He has tremendous eloquence – his father was a journalist and he inherited his gift. And, of course, he was the pioneer of liver transplantation.

Starzl was born and raised in Iowa, in the American Midwest. He then trained in a number of institutions, but the hard school of surgical apprenticeship was too soft for him. He always drove himself much more severely than was required, and he is still like this. I am told it is not easy to work for Starzl because he expects at least half as much energy from his juniors as he has himself.

I first met Starzl when he was a young surgeon in charge of the Veterans' Administration Hospital in Denver. Then we both attended a meeting in Washington DC, in 1962, with his boss, Bill Waddel. We went back to Waddel's suite of rooms in his hotel, and Starzl showed us his results. It was the first time I had seen flow charts recording the day-to-day condition of a patient in tabular form – a most important advance which enabled us to see trends occurring in different aspects of the function of the graft and behaviour of the patient. At that time Starzl was a chain-smoker, and in front of him there was a huge ashtray containing a pyramid of half-smoked, dead cigarettes.

Joseph Murray, Ken Porter and I were astonished by the detail in his report. Clearly he had obtained excellent results in kidney transplantation using the combination of azathioprine and steroids; and he personally supervised every aspect of all his patients' care.

It was less than a year later that Starzl performed the first surgically successful human liver transplant. It was a huge operation, and in those days little was known of the physiological and metabolic consequences of taking out a liver and grafting a new liver partially damaged by lack of blood supply. So Starzl's success was a very prestigious feat. Porter and I visited Starzl at this time. We arrived at Denver around ten p.m. after a long flight, and were both exhausted. When Starzl greeted us, he immediately explained that he was anxious to have Ken's opinion on some slides set up in the laboratory (Ken and he were old friends). He dragged a jet-lagged Porter off to the laboratory, where they spent the next four hours going through hundreds of slides. I excused myself and went to bed.

With such an intense and unusual character as Starzl's, anecdotes about him inevitably abounded. On one occasion Starzl was invited to a surgical meeting in Los Angeles as an honoured guest. Bad weather prevented his aeroplane from taking off in Denver, leaving dozens of surgeons waiting in vain for his speech. However, the host looked round and saw that a number of those present had worked with Starzl in Denver. After telling the disappointed audience that Starzl would not be able to make it, he suggested that each of his previous residents should stand up and tell an anecdote about their time with Starzl. Apparently this was the most entertaining evening many of the doctors present had ever experienced.

I had witnessed Starzl's legendary demands on himself and others when I visited him in 1985. As I arrived he handed me a fifty-page manuscript and asked me for my opinion. I worked hard and gave him some suggestions. The next day he looked at the suggestions and at five o'clock he asked his secretary to retype it. She took the manuscript and started typing. We went out to get something to eat and in the middle of dinner his senior assistant, Dr Shun Iwatsuki, suggested that we should get a hamburger and coffee to take back to his secretary. He handed the food to her. She was looking very tired but still typing and Starzl said, 'When will it be ready?'

'In the morning,' she replied.

At seven o'clock the next morning we went into the office. The secretary staggered forward, exhausted but smiling and handed him the completed manuscript! I asked her if she would like a job in Cambridge.

Further evidence comes from Peter Bell, Professor of Surgery in Leicester, who worked for Starzl in the late 1960s. Apparently he arrived in the department in a three-piece suit, only to find that everybody was wearing sneakers, shorts and T-shirts, and smoking. So he put away his suit and adopted the uniform. About a year later Bell had to give a paper at an important meeting so he put on his suit, but the trousers immediately fell to the ground – he had lost 3 stone in weight trying to fulfil the demanding requirements of Dr Starzl!

Starzl's pioneering of experimental and then clinical liver transplantation was his most spectacular and important achievement but, as I have already mentioned, he was also the first to keep records showing the progress of patients and to use corticosteroids in a systematic way. In addition he performed many important studies on the metabolism of the liver and the way in which a damaged liver could regenerate itself.

In Denver in the 1960s, Starzl's team was also making anti-lymphocyte globulin (ALG) as a biological treatment for rejection. This involved injecting human lymphocytes into horses; and the surgical laboratories had their own fields with horses producing the precious globulin in their blood. The technicians had to be skilful horsemen to manage the animals and collect blood for processing.

By 1968, Starzl had a small series of cases of liver grafting with a few successes, but most of his patients had died. As a result, surgeons around the world watched the Denver experience without enthusiasm. In 1967 we had developed a technique of liver transplantation and had some interesting findings on the immunology of liver grafts in pigs. I was undeterred by the orthodox, anti-transplant view and felt the time had come to embark on a clinical programme of liver transplantation of my own.

Children and Grandchildren

At this stage in our lives Patsy had a hard time raising our children on little cash, with a husband whom she saw seldom and who was usually exhausted when she did. However, she has always liked little children and this probably explains why we eventually had six. We had Debbie (born in 1962), Suzie (born in 1963) and Russell (born in 1964, and named after Russell Brock – by then Lord Brock) in London. Then, when we moved to Cambridge, after a five-year gap, Richard was born prematurely and fought hard to survive in the incubator. We felt it wiser at first not to give him a name and we called him Blob, but then, as his personality asserted itself, he became little Richard the Lionheart. We were grateful for the marvellous care he received at Addenbrooke's Hospital.

We have tried not to influence our children in their choice of profession. Nevertheless three of them have chosen to pursue careers in medicine and science. Jane studied medicine at Clare College, Cambridge, and King's College Hospital in London; Sarah studied biology at the University of East Anglia and became a teacher; Debbie studied history of art in London and works for the BBC; and Suzie trained as a nurse at the Royal Free Hospital, became an intensive care nurse and then took a degree in healthcare studies at Oxford Brookes University. She did well, gaining a first, and now edits a medical and nursing magazine, *Wound Care.* Russell is a manager responsible for planning and laying of fibreoptic communication cables, while Richard took after his grandfather and studied car engineering at Loughborough.

With the exception of Debbie, each of the children spent a formative year in Australia and we were worried that they would want to stay, but they all came back. We are now very fortunate: four of our children live in Cambridge and two in Norwich, so we meet frequently for family meals and celebrations. During their growing up years, they understood the nature of my work and this helped us through the bad as well as the good times. The four girls and Richard are married and we have five much-loved grandchildren.

Chapter Eight
Crossing the Rubicon

As anyone knows if they have read the numerous newspaper articles about liver transplants, this operation has always been a major challenge. Patients with liver failure or in the last stages of fatal liver disease will die unless the function of the diseased liver is replaced; and in some liver disorders and diseases, such as tumours, the old liver must also be removed. Replacement, in the correct (or orthotopic) position is usually best, in any case, because the liver is the largest organ in the body and is irregularly shaped and difficult to fit into the abdomen as an extra organ in an abnormal (or heterotopic) site.

The Early Days of Liver Transplantation

Thomas Starzl and Francis Moore, both working independently, had found that liver transplantation was not only a major procedure surgically, it was also extremely shocking to the recipient. In dogs and pigs there needed to be some method of bypassing the blood that is dammed up when the main vein in the body (the vena cava) and the main vein to the liver draining the intestines (the portal vein) are clamped; otherwise acute heart failure occurs. In humans, however, and especially in patients with long-standing liver disease, there are venous channels that allow temporary clamping of the major vessels. This finding was a welcome surprise. Nevertheless, as I said in the last chapter, most of the early cases resulted in the death of the patient and bereavement of the family.

There were many aspects of technique and anaesthetic care that still had to be worked out. We also needed a large infrastructure of superb intensive care nursing after the operation, and support from radiology, bacteriology, blood transfusion and biochemistry laboratories.

My own interest in liver transplantation had started when I observed that the liver was less likely to be rejected than other organs. Of course, in humans a transplanted liver will be rejected, making immunosuppression necessary, but rejection of the liver in humans was easier to control than rejection of other organ grafts. In any immunosuppressed patient with an organ graft there is a danger of sepsis, or infection, and this was in fact the cause of failure in many of the early cases performed in Cambridge. As Starzl wrote in *Annals of Surgery* (1994):

> Once a seam is opened in the fabric of the finished transplant product by rejection or by the drugs used to control it – whether this be in the graft vasculature, drainage system or any other component of the operation – the deadly handmaid of sepsis . . . is close by.

Securing drainage of bile was another major problem: if bile leaks from the duct junction, it is very irritant and liable to cause infection. It also causes fibrous scarring that blocks the passage of bile, utlimately leading to jaundice. The drainage of bile is still one of the problems plaguing liver transplantation.

Over time, however, attention to detail and learning from bitter experience were rewarded by an improvement in results, and patients could be referred for liver transplantation when they were invalids but not yet in a moribund state.

The remarkable recovery of some patients after this operation, to full and active employment and enjoyment of life, has been a great source of satisfaction to all of us involved in organ transplantation; but the dreadful disappointments in the early days led to some heart-rending scenes, and hardly left us unaffected. I remember taking the hand of a patient about to be anaesthetised for a liver graft to reassure her, and she smiled at me and said, 'Don't look so worried, Professor Calne, I'll be all right.' And she was. She gave me more confidence than I gave her.

In the 1960s, our experiments with liver grafting involved both the orthotopic operation and the insertion of an extra liver or part of a liver, called an accessory or heterotopic (meaning abnormally positioned) graft. The orthotopic operation was a better procedure in experimental animals, but there was a psychological reluctance to remove a human patient's liver, even if it was terribly diseased, since that meant the Rubicon had been crossed, and there was no going back.

While my work with pigs at the start of my stay at Addenbrooke's showed that organ graft acceptance between unrelated individuals was possible without immunosuppressive treatment, Moore's work in Boston and Starzl's in Denver had both shown that dogs did reject liver grafts. Starzl's clinical transplants in humans also behaved like liver grafts in dogs rather than pigs. Because I'd been able to demonstrate tolerance with liver grafts in pigs, I wondered if it might be easier to prevent rejection of liver grafts in man than it had been with kidney grafts.

New and dangerous operations in humans, even for dreadful, invariably fatal diseases, are not in general welcomed by the medical profession. Some 400 years ago the Italian statesman and writer Niccolò Machiavelli wrote, in another context:

> There is nothing more difficult to take in hand, more perilous to conduct, or more uncertain in its success than the introduction of a new order of things, because the innovator has for enemies all those who have done well under the old conditions and lukewarm defenders in those who may do well under the new.

In many ways medicine is as political a realm as the Medici courts from which Machiavelli was so famously barred.

The Moment of Truth

In 1968 a lady with a primary malignant growth in her liver was referred to me. She was anxious to go through this new and experimental operation, even when we had explained the numerous dangers; she said she had nothing to lose. Most of my colleagues at Addenbrooke's were opposed to my doing a liver graft for a variety of reasons.

Then, on 2 May 1968, a child with a viral brain infection became comatose, with irreversible destruction of the brain-stem. The ventilator was to be turned off, but the parents gave permission for the kidneys and liver to be used to help other patients in need.

I convened a meeting of colleagues to discuss the case. That morning, Francis Moore phoned me. By extraordinary good fortune, he happened to be in Cambridge visiting his son, a graduate student in molecular biology. I quickly asked Moore to join our meeting.

When the details of both the recipient and potential donor had been presented, I asked each of my colleagues for an opinion. They were unanimous in opposing the operation, each with a different argument – the illness of the recipient, the youth of the donor, the possibility of the donor's disease spreading to the recipient, the operation never having been done in our hospital (or even Europe) before, the prohibitive expense. After listening to this litany of pessimism, I introduced Dr Moore, world-famous (even in Cambridge), and, together with Starzl, one of the pioneers of liver grafting.

Moore's response was short and typical of him. 'Roy, you have to do it.' The opposition collapsed, and we made immediate plans for the surgery. With Moore as my first assistant, we began a long and, at that time, very difficult operation. Yet all went smoothly. I crossed the Rubicon – that is, I removed the cancerous liver in what I call the 'moment of truth', since the patient's life depends on immediate function of the new liver. As the donor was a child, the main vein draining the liver and the lower half of the body, the inferior vena cava (IVC), was very small, and I was worried that it had insufficient calibre for the adult recipient. I therefore left the

IVC in the recipient intact and joined the end of the donor IVC to the side of that of the recipient, in what came to be known as the 'piggy-back operation'. This operation was reinvented years later by other teams, who had not read our 1968 report in the *British Medical Journal*.

Our patient woke up shortly after the end of the operation, and she and we were delighted. Sadly, two and a half months later she developed a fatal pneumonia, due to the immunosuppressive drugs given to prevent rejection. We had, however, demonstrated that the operation *could* be done in Addenbrooke's Hospital. Moore's simple, forthright advocacy had won the day.

Theodor Billroth, a professor of surgery in Vienna in the nineteenth century and a close friend of the composer Johannes Brahms, developed an operation for the removal of part of the stomach in patients who could not eat because of a blockage caused by cancer or peptic ulcer. Nineteen of the first twenty patients died during or shortly after the operation, but one patient survived – and showed that the operation could be done. Now, removal of part of the stomach is a routine procedure with extremely low mortality. The same is true of liver transplantation, but in the 1960s there were still high hurdles to be leapt over.

Progress in Liver Transplantation

After the first few liver transplants had been performed at Addenbrooke's it became clear to me that, since nobody on the hospital's medical side was especially interested in the liver, I would need to seek help elsewhere. An old colleague from the Royal Free Hospital, Roger Williams, had established an extremely busy and successful liver unit at King's College Hospital in London. Williams had a surgeon's eminently practical and active mindset, and was used to making decisions and acting on them; so when I contacted him he was keen to collaborate and provide medical expertise. Because he understood prognoses and realised when conventional treatment would no longer help patients, he was well qualified to refer patients for transplantation.

We planned that I would direct the surgical procedure at Addenbrooke's while he oversaw the medical side at King's. We would do the operations at both institutions, or wherever there was a donor, since the criteria of brain death had not yet been accepted and we had less time to do the donor operation.

Events would often take the following course. We would hear of a donor in another hospital, a patient on a ventilator. A doctor would have diagnosed brain-stem destruction and decided to stop the ventilator with the relatives' consent. They would also have given permission for organs to be removed for transplantation.

Williams and I meanwhile knew that the liver was extremely sensitive to a lack of blood supply, and would be damaged during the removal procedure. It required a very high degree of co-operation from doctors, nurses and the administration of the donor hospital to overcome this difficulty, and they almost always gave it. A team of surgeons would leave from Addenbrooke's, laden with special instruments and accompanied by an operating theatre nurse, a technician to cool the liver and an intensive care nurse. From King's a medical registrar would come for a stint of twenty-four hours. He or she would then be replaced by another medical registrar, until the patient was well enough to be moved to King's or to Addenbrooke's. The liver patient, very ill, or even on a mechanical ventilator with liver failure, would be taken from King's or Addenbrooke's by special ambulance to the donor hospital.

With surgical preparations all ready, the donor patient would be moved into the operating theatre. The ventilator would be turned off, as had been planned, whether or not there was to be a transplant operation. We would wait in sterile gowns, masks and gloves until the anaesthetist declared that the heart had stopped, at which point we would be galvanised into action, immediately starting the operation: the donor liver and kidneys were now devoid of circulation and delays would render them useless.

The removal of liver and kidneys without damaging them or their blood vessels is not a particularly easy operation, and it was necessary to develop the skills to perform it swiftly. Before they were removed the liver and kidneys had to be cooled by infusing cold preservation fluid through the arteries, and they needed to cool further after removal. Then they had to be packed in sterile bags surrounded by ice. Under these circumstances kidneys could be kept for twelve to twenty-four hours, but we had to transplant the liver within a mere five to eight hours.

Once we had the donor organs, the recipient would be prepared for surgery. This operation is a two-stage one. First, the diseased liver must be removed, in what is often a very difficult operation, and then the new liver must be inserted in its normal anatomical space. One of the major complicating factors is that the liver is the main manufacturer of clotting agents in the blood: chronic liver disease causes a rise in pressure in the veins of the abdomen so that they may bleed even without being touched, just from the manoeuvres involved in preparing to take out the diseased liver. The remaining blood platelets, made by the bone marrow, are rapidly consumed by the body's attempts to clot small bleeding veins. So it is not surprising that serious blood loss, and difficulties in obtaining enough blood to replenish amounts lost during an operation, were major problems in the early days of liver transplantation. In fact, liver transplantation alone used to regularly wipe out the supplies at local blood banks – a state of affairs that almost led to a cessation of the liver transplant programme.

There was no room for error in the long surgical procedure; a mistake at any stage could have been fatal for the recipient. The operation was usually accompanied by the unpleasant whirring noise of the sucker removing the blood that was shed. As soon as the sucker could be turned off safely the surgeon knew that the patient was probably out of the wood. If possible, the operation was carried out in a systematic way, one part at a time, and if bleeding occurred in one area then it was often best to leave that area temporarily and come back to it later.

Before inserting the new liver, a decision had to be made, in consultation with the anaesthetist, as to whether or not to bypass the blood from the big veins in the lower part of the body to the major draining vein in the upper part of the body. This took extra time and had its own hazards. Bypass required the expertise of a special pump technician to make sure that the blood flow through the bypass system was adequate and safely administered. It was vital no air got into the circuit, as it could be fatal.

At the end of the operation we knew the liver should look perfect, with good pulsation in the artery, a soft portal vein and soft vena cava above and below the liver, safe drainage of the bile duct to that of the recipient, and no bleeding. If everything had gone well the abdomen was then closed and the patient was returned to the intensive care ward by the anaesthetist. Occasionally, if there was severe bleeding which could not be stopped, gauze packs were inserted and left in place for forty-eight hours and then removed. This lesson had been learned from the treatment of liver trauma (see page 77). The gauze packs helped to stop the bleeding and have saved many lives over the years. The operation could take anything between just over two hours to more than twelve. The average was about three to four hours in an uncomplicated case.

For patients who survived the operation, the experience could be surreal. They might wake up in a strange hospital, having never even been to that town before. The relatives had to come long distances to visit, and it could be ten days to two weeks before the patient was well enough to be transferred back to King's or Addenbrooke's. In truth, the logistics of this arrangement were impossibly complex: the disturbance of the local hospital and the reliance on the goodwill of the staff were too much to expect except in a few exceptional institutions. But there were very few donors in our own hospitals.

All this changed when it became possible to remove organs while the donor was still on the ventilator and the circulation of the vital organs was intact. We could then remove the livers in distant hospitals and bring them back to either Addenbrooke's or King's for grafting. But, while the practicalities became easier, there was still little general enthusiasm for liver transplantation in the 1960s, and the results remained extremely poor for some time. Nevertheless the dramatic successes we achieved, however few in number, convinced us that the procedure was possible and worthwhile. When a life-saving operation, despite an extremely high early mortality, is shown to be possible, it eventually becomes established, the errors are recognised and eliminated, and a new generation of surgeons wonders why the pioneers had such a hard time.

Two Early Successes

Mrs Winnie Smith was referred to me around this time. She had a large liver tumour involving both sides of the liver, so it could not be removed and leave her with enough liver to support life. She was a plump, cheerful lady of forty-eight, living in the nearby town of Welwyn with her husband and two children, and worked as a hospital cleaner. We discussed the option of a liver transplant and she was keen to go ahead with it. The weather was deteriorating and heavy snow was falling when a road traffic accident victim suffering from brain damage was admitted to Newmarket hospital, fourteen miles from Cambridge.

As I have explained, in those days we used to move the recipient to the donor hospital, so in this case our surgical team went to Newmarket and Mrs Smith was admitted there. The operation was long but went well and one of our surgeons stayed to take care of her. She made a good recovery and when the snow melted she was transferred to Addenbrooke's and later discharged. She went back to work and taking care of her family.

When the International Transplantation Society Meeting was held in San Francisco in 1972 I managed to raise funds so that Mrs Smith could go. She came, accompanied by her husband, and they found their first trip abroad a most exciting experience. Her case was presented and she took the platform and answered questions from the audience. At that time it was nearly five years since her transplant and she was one of the longest survivors. However, shortly after returning home she developed jaundice, due to blockage of the bile duct, which led to a fatal infection in the bloodstream. It was a sad ending for a marvellous and inspiring patient who had shown us and the world that liver transplantation really could give dying patients a new lease of life.

At the same meeting a paper was presented by W. T. Summerlin, a young scientist from the famous Sloan-Kettering Institute in New York, claiming that mouse and human skin cultured from 1–6 weeks led to their permanent survival when allografted. The presentation was received by thunderous applause and prominent members of the audience left their chairs to congratulate the speaker. Derek Samson, a colleague of mine sitting next to me, asked if I was going to join the throng around Dr Summerlin. I declined, and told Derek I did not believe the work, since Summerlin had reported 100 per cent success and such a result could never be obtained in biological systems. My disbelief was vindicated when several distinguished scientists failed to confirm Summerlin's results, and a technician riding in the lift with Dr Summerlin saw him painting a fake skin graft with a felt pen on a rat he was going to use to demonstrate his success to his boss.

Gordon Bridewell is our longest survivor with a liver graft. Here was a young man in a terrible situation, with a family history of liver disease. He had the dreaded hepatitis B virus which had caused cirrhosis of the liver, and on top of this he developed a huge tumour – also in his liver.

His brother had died from the same disease a few months previously and, as a result, Gordon turned up at King's College in a desperate state. At that time we had not defined our indications and contra-indications for liver transplantation and we were prepared to take all comers. So we did a transplant on Gordon in King's, after finding that the huge tumour on his liver had apparently not spread elsewhere. We gave him gamma globulin injections against hepatitis B, which is often not effective, but we started the treatment when his diseased liver came out and for a short period after the new liver had been inserted.

Against all the odds, he did very well. He left hospital and was soon rehabilitated and back at work as a car engineer. Twenty-three years later, when he was knocked off his bicycle by a lorry and developed pain over ribs that had been fractured, there was concern that he might have damaged his liver transplant. However, he recovered from this added injury and it transpired that we had a shared interest in painting – I did a portrait of Gordon and he presented me with a painting of the West Country where he lived. While he was sitting for the portrait he asked me a very pertinent question: 'If I came to see you now with the condition I was suffering from twenty-three years ago, I don't think you'd accept me for a transplant, would you?' The truthful answer, which was the one I gave him, was that no, we would not.

He had two major contra-indications to a liver transplant, hepatitis B and the large tumour which we would have expected to recur. So he is the exception which proves the rule – our longest survivor with a liver transplant, still at work now, nearly twenty-five years after the operation. He taught us another important lesson – that we can make general assessments based on statistics but each patient is an individual, with his or her unique biological reaction to a transplant. For this reason, we can never say for certain what the outcome will be in a particular case. We can only give an overall statistical impression of what would be expected to happen, according to our experience of liver transplantation in our own unit and worldwide.

Under the Sword of Damocles

For reasons already mentioned, we used a vast amount of blood in nearly all the early liver transplant operations. A complicating factor was that the blood bank would not issue extra blood clotting factors unless there was a demonstrable defect in the specimens we had sent to the laboratory. Because there was a time lag between collecting the blood, sending it to the laboratory and getting the result, the patient could deteriorate to a critical state during this time, losing blood, consuming the few clotting factors that were left and producing the usually fatal condition we call 'red ink syndrome', when the blood fails to clot successfully.

I asked for clotting factors urgently for a patient in this condition, and was told by the haematology lab that the clotting factors in the sample of the patient's blood were normal. The patient was meanwhile losing copious amounts of blood onto the floor. I spoke to the consultant haematologist and said that perhaps if she came to the operating theatre, she would be convinced that their assessment was erroneous. She reluctantly said she would come, but didn't know which theatre we would be in. I explained that this would be a very easy task for her: all she had to do was walk along the corridor, and enter the operating theatre with a pool of blood issuing from beneath the door. She came and was suitably impressed, realising that the arrangements for blood clotting were unsatisfactory. So together we worked out a method of assessing blood clotting in the operating theatre and giving clotting factors before, rather than after, the patient had lost vast quantities of blood.

Thus within a relatively short period of time we were able to remove the anxieties over blood supplies that had hung like the sword of Damocles over the whole liver transplantation programme. Today we still sometimes require large volumes of blood, up to 50 or even 100 units, but usually we require less than 10 units and occasionally none at all.

One special case was a young boy from a family of Jehovah's Witnesses. Oddly, Jehovah's Witnesses permit transplantation of organs, which, of course, always contain blood, but do not permit in any way a blood transfusion – not even taking blood from the patient, storing it and giving it back. This presents a certain challenge for the doctor, and in fact the parents who brought their boy to see me said that they had been to all the liver transplant units in Britain, and nobody would do a liver transplant unless they had permission to use blood. I explained that to start such a procedure, which nearly always requires some blood, and see a young boy die just because a few units of blood were needed and couldn't be given, would have a disastrous effect on the nursing and medical team: it was not reasonable to expect them to proceed in this way. Nevertheless, I said, I would try not to use blood but I wouldn't start the operation unless I had their permission to give blood *in extremis.*

The boy's parents reluctantly agreed to this and the anaesthetist was extremely careful, as were we on the surgical side. Blood substitutes were given, and at the end of the operation the patient was in good condition with a new liver, and no blood had been used. The parents were delighted, and every year I receive a card telling me that the boy is doing well and they are so grateful that no blood was needed.

Hair-raising Journeys

In the early days of transplantation blood supply was not our only problem; the sheer hard slog of getting the organs was a never-ending trial. Since donors were scarce, I would travel long distances to acquire livers for my patients, sometimes with a surgical nurse, technician and surgical assistant. We would take off in a small plane or helicopter from the playing field beside Addenbrooke's and fly to the donor, remove the liver, come back, and start the transplant operation. From start to finish, the whole procedure might take more than thirty-six hours – an exhausting, punishing regimen – but it was a remarkable team, and they all continued to support liver transplantation through those difficult years. Patsy would act as unpaid coordinator, contacting by phone the many people who needed to be informed.

These journeys could be dramatic, and not just because of the urgency of our mission. The flights themselves, while often invigorating, could also be terrifying. One Christmas Eve we were on a night flight to Manchester, and were told to look out for the headlights of two police cars which would illuminate the landing point for our helicopter. The pilot was having difficulty determining exactly where we were, when suddenly he saw the headlights of two police cars and started to descend. Sitting next to the pilot, I noticed out of the corner of my eye a pylon and electricity wire directly beneath us. I literally screamed this information to the pilot who, just in time, moved the helicopter back up in a lunge to a safe position. A fraction of a second later, and we'd have been destroyed. When we shakily approached the police cars, we found they were involved in some crime-busting operation, and 'our' police cars were in fact parked several miles away.

Another memorable trip was in a military helicopter rather like a cattle truck, which was fearfully noisy on take-off, and very cold in the winter too. We had to set off for Bristol, but in the middle of a snowstorm which made visibility dreadful. The pilot decided that we could not reach Bristol and would land at the RAF base near Oxford. With extreme aplomb – and accuracy – he landed on the lawn outside the commanding officer's residence, which he said he was permitted to do in emergency conditions. Then he took out a little case which contained his service uniform. It just so happened that he knew there was a big full-dress party in the mess that night and he had arranged for invitations for all of us too.

After an enjoyable evening, we continued our journey at the crack of dawn, and, once again, the pilot had difficulty with navigation. This time he decided on an unusual method: he followed a road until we reached a crossroads and a traffic sign; he then hovered over the sign, and a terrified and rather astonished car driver, until we had deciphered the direction of Bristol. With renewed confidence we continued on our way. The liver was removed without trouble and we headed back home.

But our tribulations weren't over. In the middle of southern England is a conglomeration of electrical power cables and pylons, so convoluted that the air crew of our helicopter used it as an obstacle course for training. The warrant officer opened the door of the 'cattle truck' and, leaning out with a rope around him, shouted instructions to the pilot while the helicopter hovered a few feet above the top of the live wires, then dipped down to go beneath the wires of the next pylon. The air crew much enjoyed this leap-frogging, rather like tracing a purl stitch in knitting, and they performed the manoeuvre many times with extreme accuracy and confidence. We were utterly terrified – not to mention half-frozen, because the door was open. It was a great relief when we continued on to Cambridge.

We also flew in aeroplanes – commercial aircraft, but more often privately hired small planes, usually with a pilot and navigator, and sometimes just a pilot. On one occasion in 1979 we were invited to the Netherlands to remove a liver from a young girl who had tragically died following cardiac bypass surgery. We flew to

Schiphol Airport, proceeded to the hospital and then, when the liver was removed, were escorted back to the airport by an unrequested posse of police motorcycles. First one policeman arrived, then two, then four. The cavalcade screamed through the streets and along the motorway, arriving at the airport only to find that the pilot was having his lunch and we had to wait another twenty minutes.

Nor was this the end of the drama. On arriving at Heathrow, we were bundled into a police car, a Rover V8, to get to King's. The journey, which would normally take the best part of an hour, was accomplished in twenty minutes with sirens and flashing lights, terrorising citizens who happened to be on the same route. On arrival at King's, the Rover came to an abrupt standstill, and there was a tremendous explosion as the radiator top came off and boiling water shot up in a rust-coloured fountain at the front of the car. Our technician, who had been holding the liver, also 'exploded', to her great embarrassment: the final shock caused her to empty her bladder. We all had to calm down before getting started on the transplant operation.

On another occasion I was called back from Paris to do a liver transplant at Addenbrooke's. A special single-engine plane was sent for me but the weather was rapidly deteriorating and the pilot told me that we were going to have a bad journey because there was a thunderstorm over the Channel. His prediction was correct: the little plane lurched to and fro in the storm, and I saw, to my horror, purple light flickering around the windscreen. The pilot dismissed it as an electrostatic disturbance, common in a thunderstorm, and actually seemed to be enjoying the trip. I was exhausted and relieved to land at Heathrow, and even pleased to continue the journey in a police car, this time driving just fast.

Sensational as these trips were, they pale beside the experience of a team in Scotland, who managed to drop a liver out of a helicopter into the Firth of Forth near Edinburgh – amazingly, without harming the organ, which was retrieved in good condition for transplantation.

In fact, with all the rushing around that went into the early development of organ transplantation and the hundreds of thousands of transplants that have been performed, it is remarkable that not a single fatal accident has occurred in connection with the procedure.

The Logistics of Liver Transplantation

Despite all the work Roger Williams and I, and our teams, put into the venture, our liver transplant programme was not initially granted a budget. It was not even considered by the administration as a distinct unit: it just seemed to fit in, as a variant of the reasonably well-established kidney programme. It gradually became apparent, however, that liver transplantation was an expensive exercise, involving intensive care beds, blood requirements, personnel, and of course the chartering of flights to destinations as far away as Scotland or southern Europe. So the situation began to change.

Now there are seven liver transplantation units in Britain, budgeted directly from the Treasury via the Department of Health. In order to reduce costs, each unit has been assigned a geographical zone within which it is responsible for removing organs for transplantation. The liver and kidney units trust each other to remove the organs in good condition for transplanting in another centre – a degree of trust that has not yet permeated to the cardiac transplanters. The most efficient method of organ removal, however, is for a single team to be responsible for the removal of both thoracic and abdominal organs. This means that fewer people are needed and the disturbance of the donor hospital is reduced. There must be a fair distribution of organs to each individual centre, since the removal is hard work, usually taking place in the middle of the night, and always involving the tragedy of bereaved relatives, which has a traumatic effect on the doctors and nurses in the donor hospital.

Unlike kidney transplants, in which there is no doubt that grafting between blood relatives gets better results than between unrelated individuals, such a tissue match does not seem to hold in liver transplants. In fact, in some diseases where there is an auto-immune process (such as biliary cirrhosis), the better the tissue match, the worse the results. In kidney transplantation there is continual negotiation between surgeons who want an organ removed as expeditiously as possible with the minimal period of storage and transportation, and tissue-typing immunologists who feel that getting a good tissue type is more important than speed.

Paul Terasaki, one of the doyens of tissue-typing, has shown that transplantation of kidneys between non-related individuals – usually husband to wife or wife to husband – gets results that are as good as those between parents and children. This is a strong argument for ensuring that organs for transplantation have minimal damage from removal and storage, even at the expense of accepting a less good tissue match.

A Trip to China

In the summer of 1970 came the first of my three trips to China. I was approached by the Ministry of Health and asked if I would be prepared to take a delegation to China to lecture on liver transplantation and demonstrate operations. I gathered that there had been some disagreement between our ambassador in Peking, Chinese health officials and our own Department of Health as to whether liver transplantation was an appropriate subject for a visit to a developing country such as China. However, I was glad that the Chinese prevailed and we had a chance to go there. Our mission was to visit centres in China where there was interest in liver transplantation and discuss the subject with our Chinese colleagues. They particularly wanted us to instruct them in the properties of the new immunosuppressant, cyclosporin, which we had developed in the laboratory and had been the first to use in clinical transplantation.

China at this time had recently emerged from the black era of the Cultural Revolution and all the Chinese we met were jubilant about having 'smashed the Gang of Four' who they claimed were responsible for the disaster. The human and cultural destruction caused by the Cultural Revolution still affects China today. A whole generation of students was deprived of education, and a whole nation's traditional respect for learning was jettisoned by a wave of the elderly, crazed Mao's hand. Professors, artists, musicians and poets were beaten; many were killed; others were driven to suicide. The lucky ones were banished thousands of miles away to the country to work as serfs for the farmers. It was extraordinary that such things could happen in a country with traditions of civilisation going back thousands of years. In 1970 the doors of China were just starting to be cautiously opened to the West.

Our team consisted of myself; Dr Mike Lindop, the anaesthetist; Sister Celia Chan, a Singaporean/Cantonese/Chinese theatre sister; and Michael Smith, senior operating department assistant and technician. We were in fact a very modest and benign 'Gang of Four', despatched economy class to Hong Kong where we were housed at the YMCA. For me it was particularly interesting to return to Hong Kong after my days there in the army. It had changed almost beyond recognition – an enormous number of new buildings had appeared and the economy was booming. At night the streets were brightly lit with neon advertisements, but, whatever is done to Hong Kong, the harbour and Peak Mountain will always remain beautiful.

We were entertained by friends of my family, Dr and Mrs David Kwok, who took us all over the island, Kowloon and the New Territories, where we were able to sample wonderful Chinese meals. After a few days in Hong Kong we took the train to Canton and then travelled in an old China Airways trident to Peking. Having a Cantonese and Mandarin-speaking team member was a huge advantage, making it very difficult for the political liaison officers to pull the wool over our eyes.

At Peking Medical College the buildings were so cold that we had to wear our overcoats indoors. We found that factory workers were paid considerably more than nurses, and doctors received only a little more than factory workers. As with the animals in George Orwell's *Animal Farm*, so in China all people were equal but some more equal than others. For example, the party members had beautiful worsted suits (admittedly in the Mao style) whereas most people had to make do with rough material.

Bureaucracy apparently existed in China before Christ but it was certainly flourishing under the Communists. Even simply changing money required six steps: a man came with a form that had to be filled in; another man carried the form to a girl; the girl recorded the form in a book; a man took the form to the cashier; the cashier got the money out; and the man took the money from the cashier back to the customer. Even with the proliferation of managers in British hospitals in recent years and the vast increase in bureaucracy, we are still relative novices at this. We could learn a great deal from the Chinese when it comes to complicating matters further with no advantage to anyone.

The Chinese hospital operating theatres were, by our standards, primitive (to put it mildly). Blood transfusions were given in an open flask with muslin over the top, and the blood was poured into the muslin. Acupuncture was not very popular in surgery, since they had found that many patients were unsusceptible to it. The Chinese anaesthetists usually preferred to use Western drugs, but we did see a thyroid removed under acupuncture. Alcohol was frowned upon by the authorities but we met many youngsters who seemed to enjoy both beer and the extremely powerful liquor called Maotai, which in its rough form smells and tastes like petrol. After the wonderful food we had had in Hong Kong the food in China was dreadful, mainly due to a shortage of basic ingredients. We subsisted on a diet of sweet-and-sour fat, cabbage soup and rice.

We travelled to Wuhan, where there was a tradition of experimental and clinical organ grafting, and we demonstrated liver transplantation experimentally. The intensive care ward was a concrete yard outside the hospital. Of course the Chinese are technically brilliant and very studious and knowledgeable; but they were working under terrible conditions, with the heavy hand of bureaucracy stifling any individual initiative. In Wuhan we met the Professor of Acupuncture who took us round his clinic. Apart from acupuncture, they also used 'cupping' (a popular form of treatment in Europe from medieval times until the eighteenth century) and moxibustion, which is a heat treatment for a painful area. In cupping, a candle is lit inside a cup which is then placed over the painful area; this exhausts the oxygen and sucks the flesh into the cup. All the conditions being treated in the clinic were similar to those that would be treated in physiotherapy clinics in the West; and, in fact, the pattern of recovery seemed very similar to that of our patients sent for physiotherapy. Most got better in time, except those with irreversible structural damage.

In Wuhan we learnt that there was no air, train or road transport available to take us to Shanghai, but that space had been booked for us on a boat on the River Yangtse. This boat trip took four days, and we stopped at many villages and towns on the way. There seemed to be thousands of people on board and many animals.

On 10 November we approached Shanghai and the weather became much warmer. A beautiful junk under full sail was tacking across the harbour and there was an array of ancient coal-burning steam ships, old dreadnoughts and cargo vessels. It was like going back to the 1930s. Mike Lindop and I played tennis and we stayed at the Jing-jaing Hotel, in the old French colonial district. The food in Shanghai was a little better than elsewhere and on one occasion we went to the famous Greenwaves Restaurant. Mike Smith, a huge man who normally enjoys his food, started his bowl of soup with reasonable enthusiasm until he saw what looked like a small dead bird floating in it among the noodles.

In Shanghai we gathered that more than 100 liver transplants had been performed in China but there wasn't one patient surviving long term. They didn't appear to have a satisfactory infrastructure and they were very reluctant to discuss organ donation. We had the impression, later confirmed, that most of the organs they used for transplantation came from criminals who had been executed.

Our last visit was to Canton, which was more influenced by the West, with large new commercial buildings and hotels and a rather surly attitude on the part of the hotel staff. In every medical school we visited, the surgeons, who had obviously received directives for their research from Peking, were performing the same experiments. Such central authority inevitably stifles new ideas.

It took only twenty-five minutes to fly back to Hong Kong from

Canton, but the contrast was amazing: from the stark, colourless Communist regime to the pulsating, money-based, over-crowded Hong Kong. My feeling at the end of the trip was that mainland China was unlikely to take over Hong Kong; more probably Hong Kong would take over China. Indeed, since the handover in 1997, it would seem that mainland China is increasingly following the commercial pattern of Hong Kong, even though the Peking regime remains extremely autocratic. The volatile financial situation in south-east Asia may yet lead to further surprises.

Chapter Nine

The Search for New Drugs

After 6MP and azathioprine, I had spent nearly twenty years searching for and testing new compounds that might prevent graft rejection. The results were usually disappointing. Then, in 1977, Jean Borel, director of the microbiology department at the pharmaceutical company, Sandoz, in Basel, Switzerland, presented to the British Society of Immunology his experiments on the cyclic peptide cyclosporin A. Derived from a malodorous fungus, this substance could, as Borel showed, prolong skin graft survival and inhibit immune reactions. David White, an immunologist in my department at Addenbrooke's, thought this compound might have an anti-macrophage action and we were at that time interested in the macrophage (the scavenger cell of the immune system). Meanwhile, one of my visiting Fellows, a Greek surgeon called Alkis Kostakis, had spent nearly two years with us, but had had no success with his experiments. Kostakis told me that his professor in Athens would be upset if he did not produce anything during his time in Cambridge. He said he wanted to study immunosuppression; so he learnt how to transplant hearts heterotopically in rats, and then started looking at conventional immunosuppressive drugs.

An Unusual Use for Olive Oil

White thought Kostakis might like to look at cyclosporin A. Two months later Kostakis came to me, very excited, describing the wonderful results he had obtained with cyclosporin in prolonging heart transplants in the rat. Kostakis related his experimental findings in the ward during the 1977 Wimbledon tennis semi-finals, which I was watching with a patient, so I only half-heard what he was telling me. Eventually he and I sat down together, and he gave me details of his experiment.

It sounded too good to be true, but on repetition even better results were obtained with a Greek solvent for cyclosporin A – best-quality olive oil that Kostakis had been sent by his mother, who was worried that he might starve in England. I phoned Sandoz, and asked for some cyclosporin A to study in large animals. They told me they had stopped working with the compound but we could have some of what was left in their lab. I went on to investigate cyclosporin A in dogs with kidney grafts and in pigs with orthotopic heart grafts. In all the experiments we carried out, we found that it was far better than any other agent, and we proceeded to plan a pilot experiment for the use of cyclosporin A in man.

However, first it was necessary for us to go to Basel, to convince the hard-headed business chiefs of Sandoz that this development was worthwhile. They somewhat reluctantly agreed, believing that developing cyclosporin would be regarded as an ethical and humanitarian gesture but would probably be a money loser. They had no idea that this compound would revolutionise organ transplantation, create a huge new market, and become a gigantic source of revenue for their company.

We at Addenbrooke's were the first to use cyclosporin A in patients with organ grafts, but it was a bumpy ride initially. To our intense worry, the early trials with patients demonstrated a completely unexpected side-effect in humans: the drug actually damaged the kidneys. None of the animal experiments had hinted at such a complication. It took some time to adjust the dose so that kidney damage could be averted, but after this had

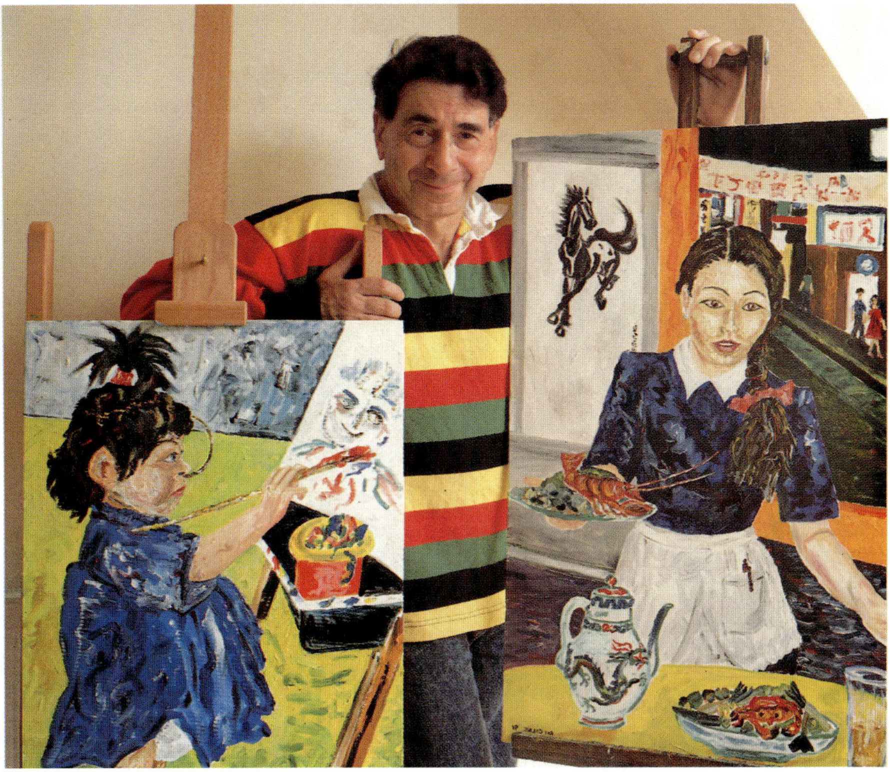

In my studio with a painting of Tamara Rainey (*left*), a brave little girl from Belfast who has had four liver transplants (*Daily Telegraph*)

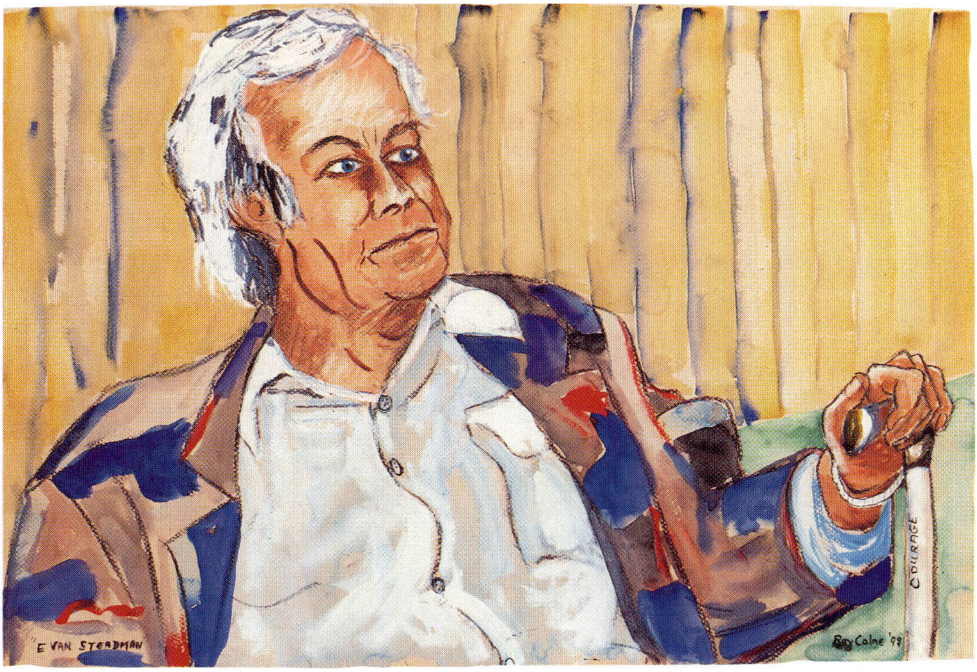

In spite of three liver transplants, sepsis and cancer, Evan Steadman amazed us all with his sheer courage and determination

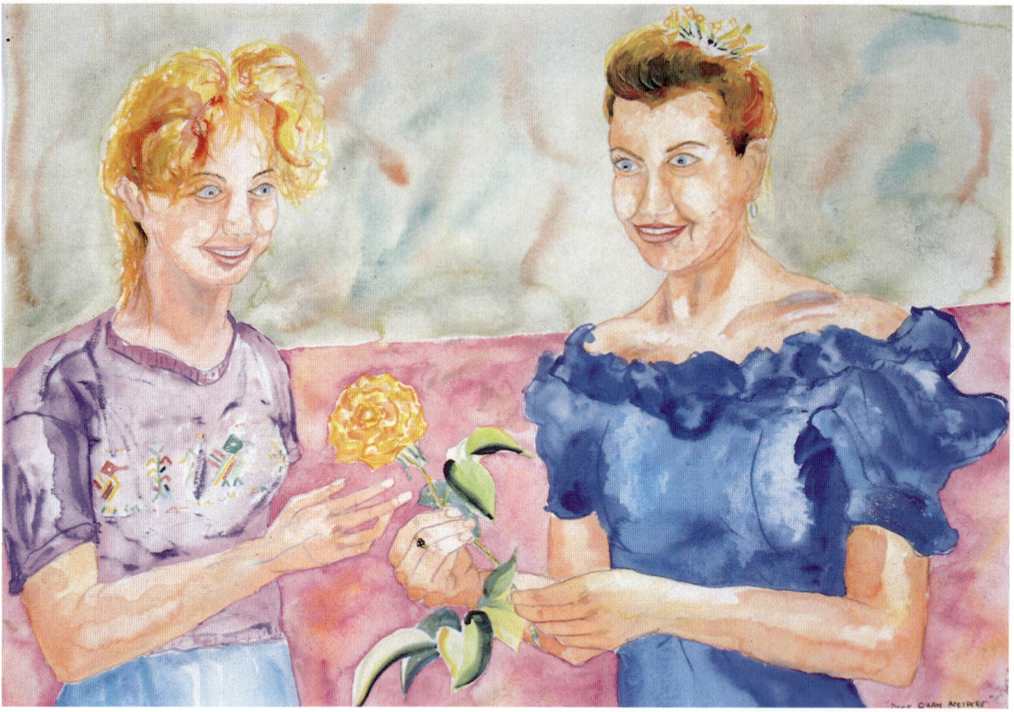

Dare quam accipere – to give rather than to receive – is the motto of Guy's Hospital where I trained. The yellow rose signifies the gift of life. The girl on the left received a kidney from the girl on the right who died in a road accident.

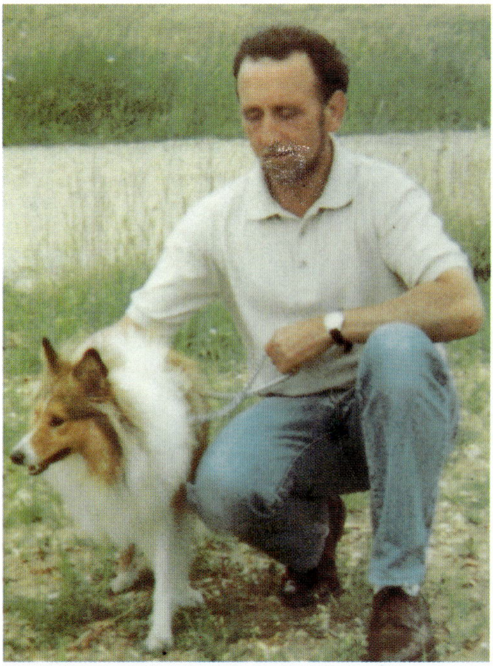

Gordon Bridewell, our longest-surviving liver transplant patient, twenty-five years after his operation

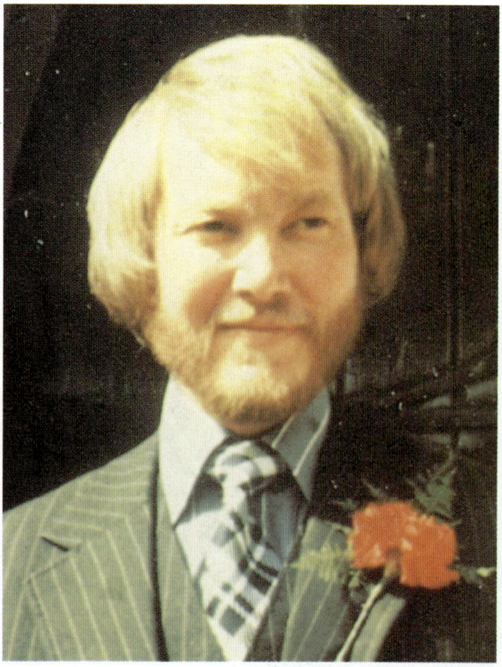

Nigel McLeod at his wedding in 1976, ten years after he received a kidney transplant from an unrelated cadaver donor. He is still well thirty-two years after his operation.

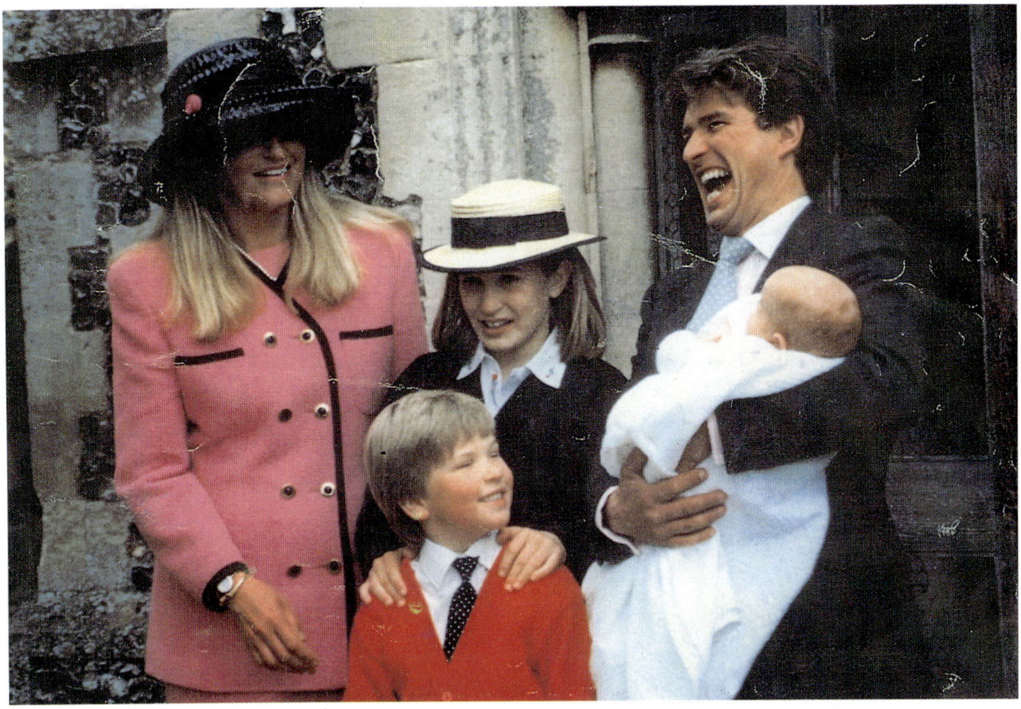

Annabel Johnson, who received a kidney from her brother, with her family

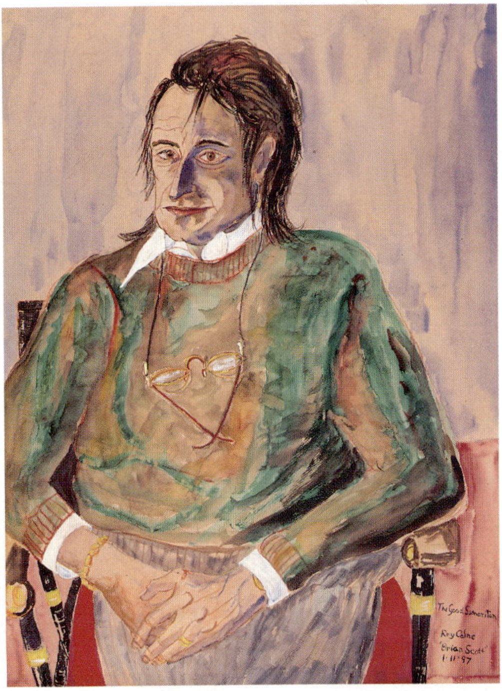

Brian Scott, the Good Samaritan, who had been attacked while helping an old lady in a New York street

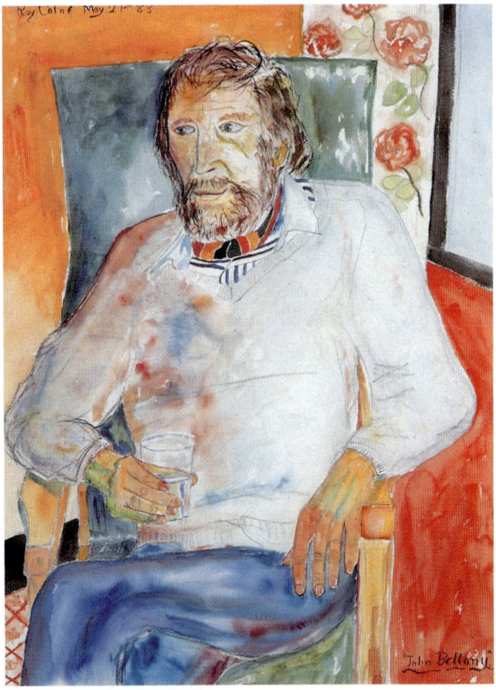

John Bellany, the distinguished Scottish painter, recovering in hospital after his liver transplant

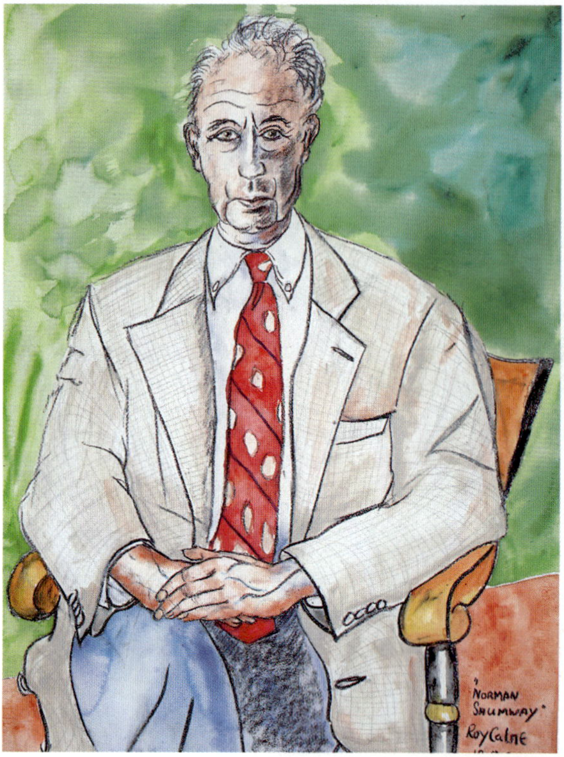

Dr Norman Shumway, one of the pioneers of heart transplantation

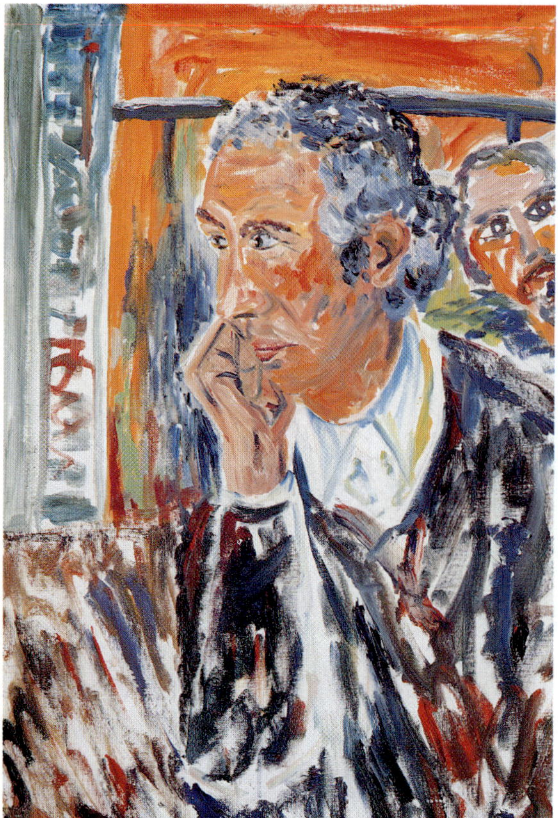

Dr Jean Borel, who discovered the immunological properties of cyclosporin – a turning point in organ transplantation

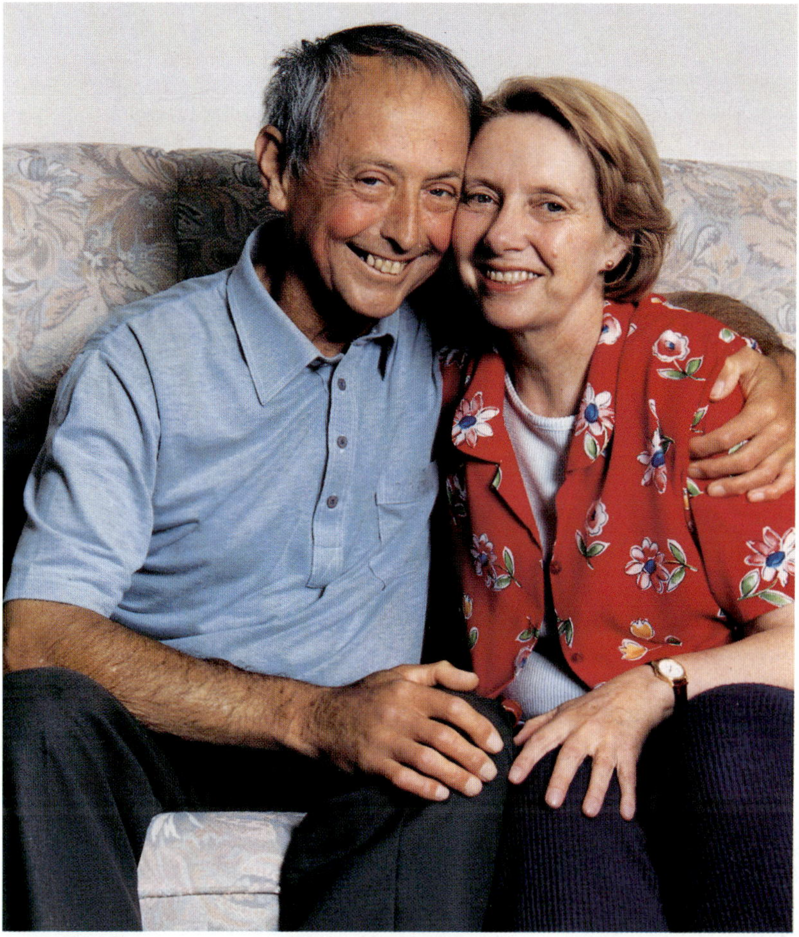

Monica Wildsmith gave a kidney to her husband Alan in the first non-related living transplant in Cambridge

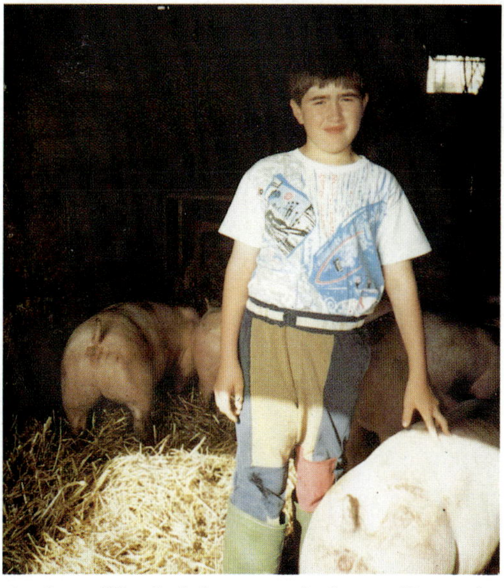

Andrew Hardwick – no relation to Ben – is now a strapping teenager, twelve years after his liver transplant

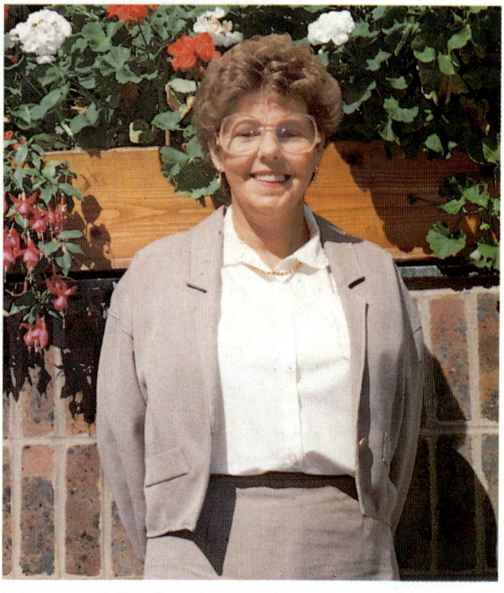

The world's first heart, lung and liver transplant patient, Davina Thompson, who sadly died twelve years after her operation.

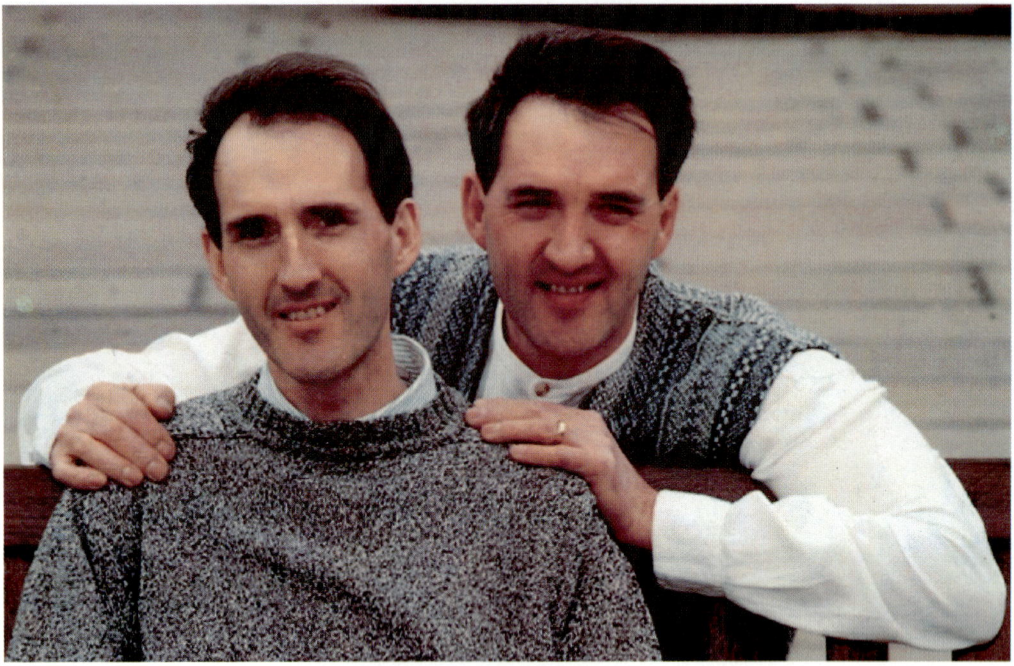

Two of the Jones identical triplets: Peter gave Philip a portion of his bowel. The graft functions normally without immunosuppression

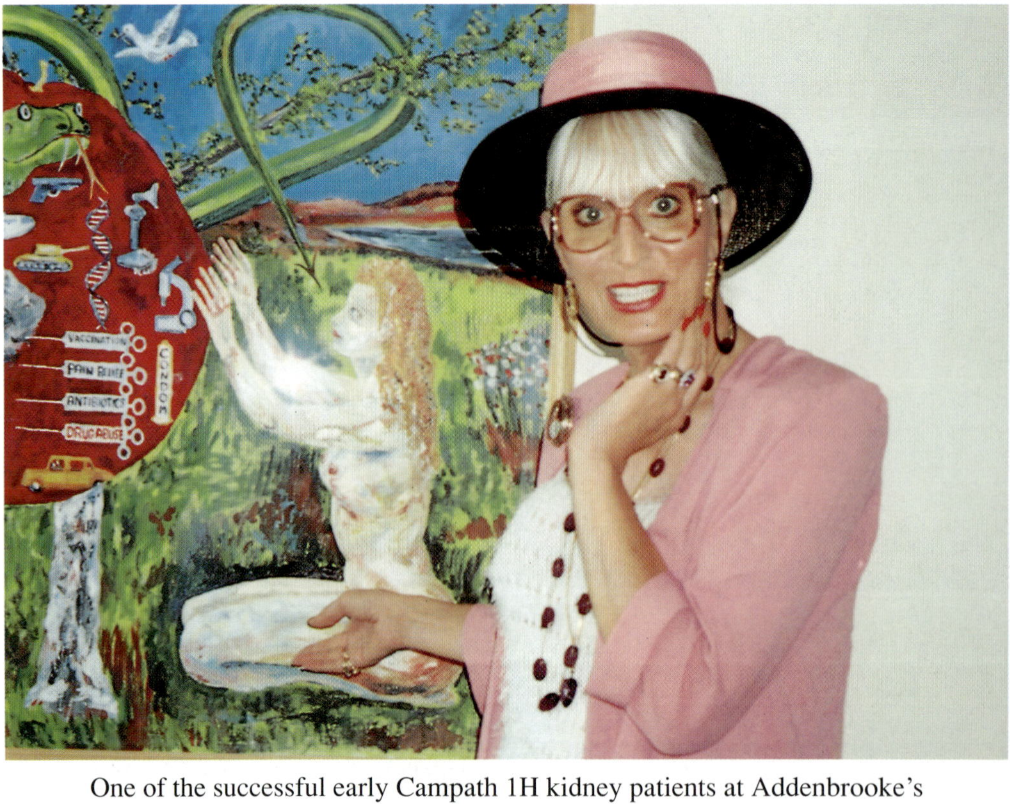

One of the successful early Campath 1H kidney patients at Addenbrooke's

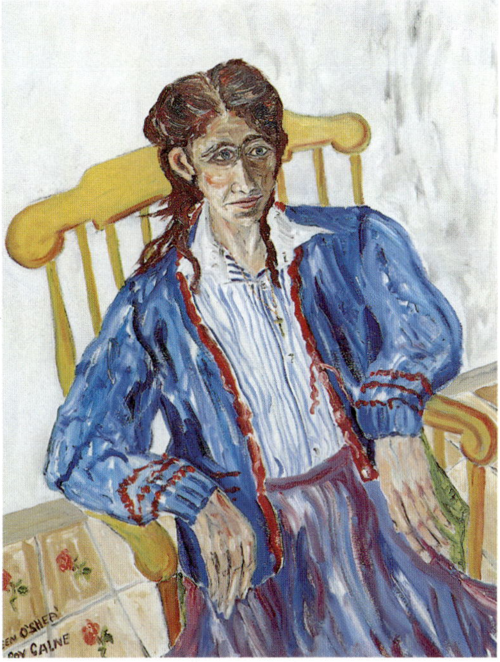
O'SHEA
ROY CALNE

Nurse Eileen O'Shea who underwent four liver transplants

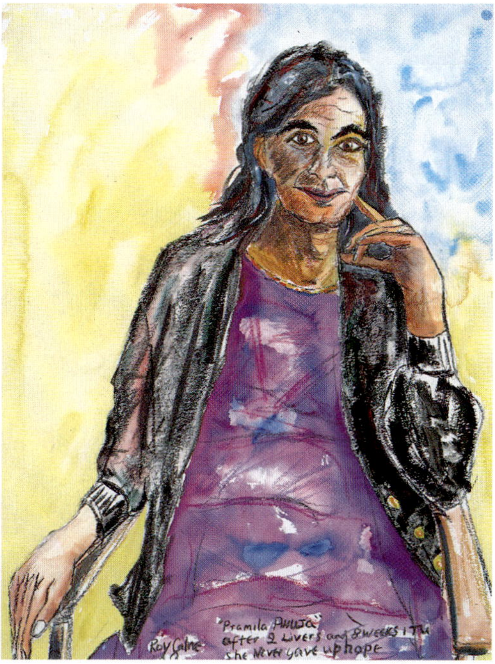
"Pramila Ahuja"
after 2 Livers and 8 WEEKS ITU
she never gave up hope
Roy Calne

Pramila Ahuja was encouraged by the words whispered to her by her hepatologist Graeme Alexander, 'Don't give up, keep on fighting, you're going to get better'

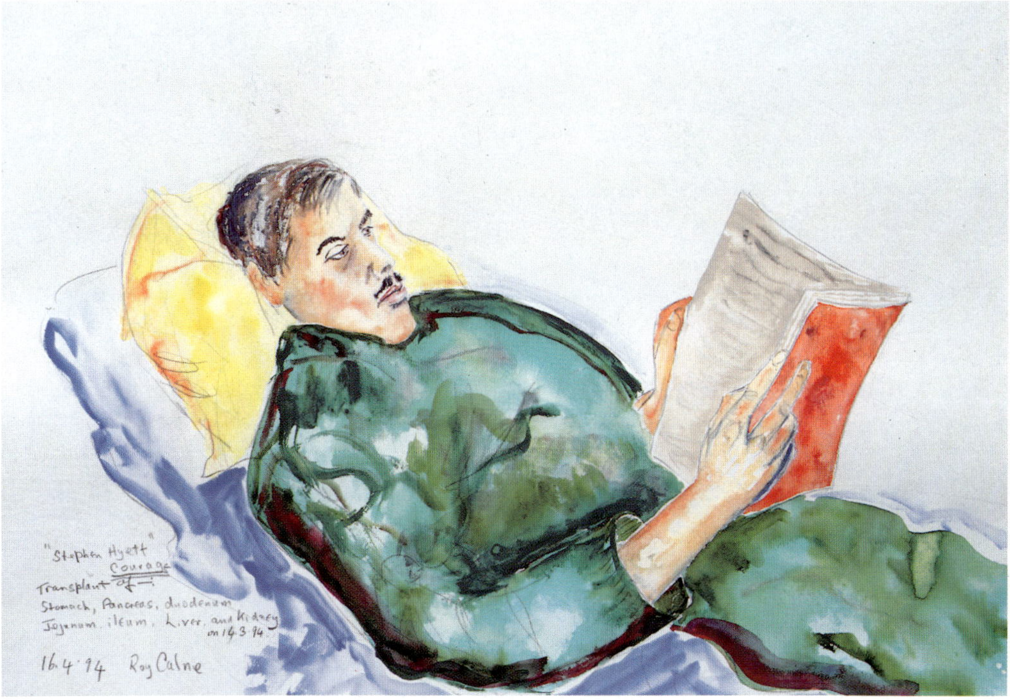
"Stephen Hyatt"
Courage
Transplant of
Stomach, Pancreas, duodenum
Jejunum, ileum, Liver, and Kidney
on 14.3.94
16.4.94 Roy Calne

Still well five years after a six-organ transplant: Stephen Hyatt received stomach, duodenum, small bowel, liver, pancreas and kidney

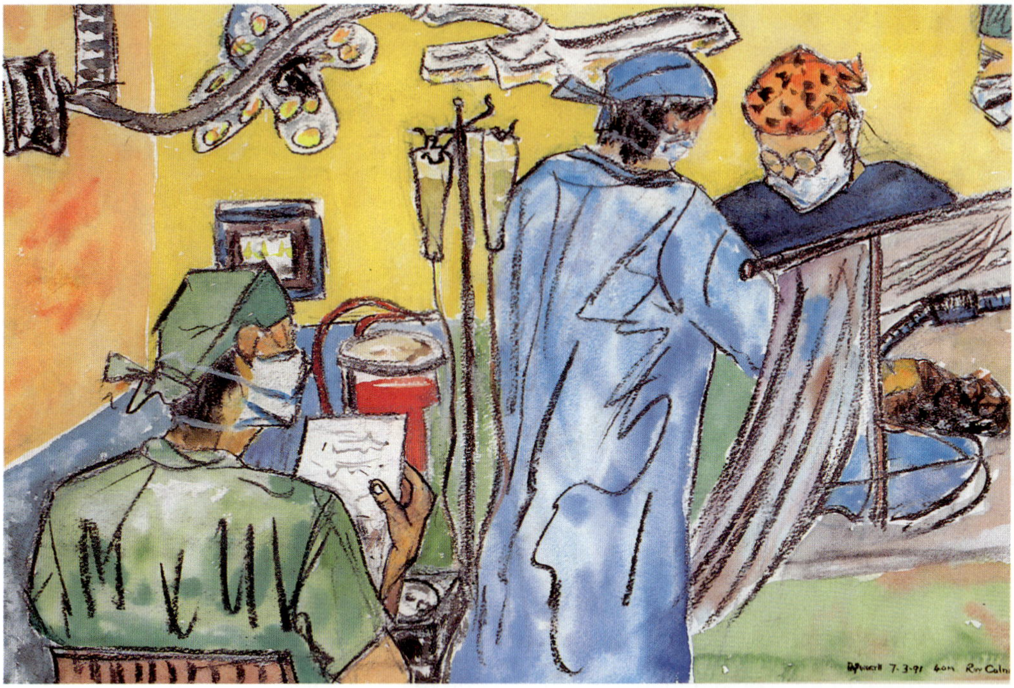

Papworth 91: an operating theatre sketch of a heart, lungs and liver transplantation in progress

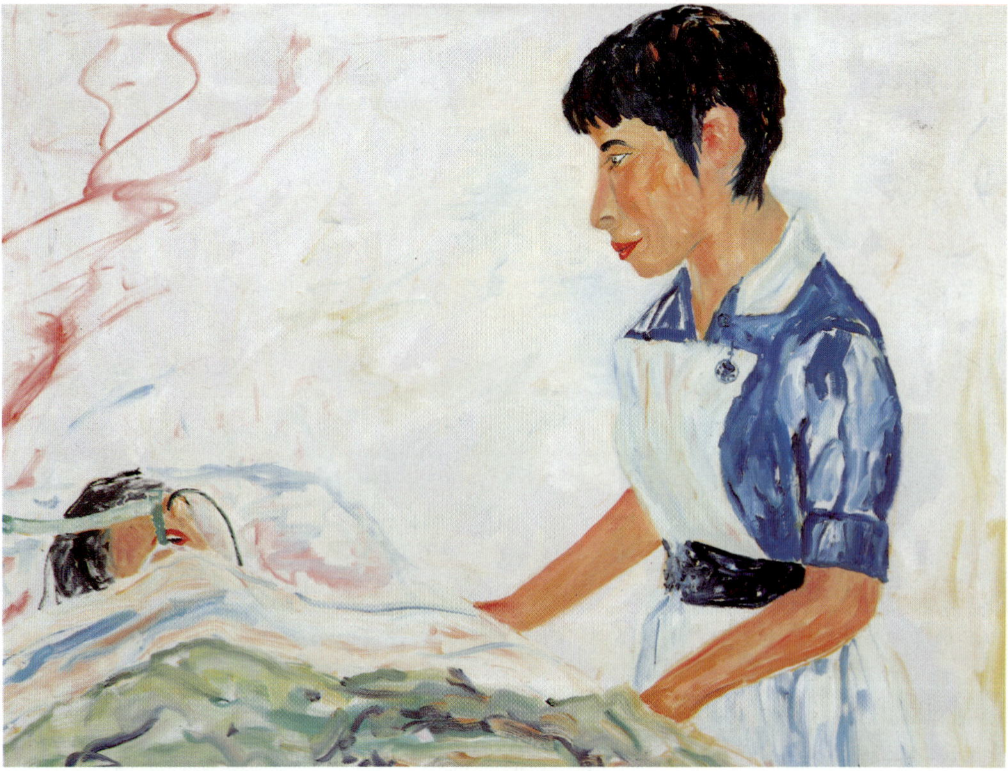

The skill and compassion of the Intensive Care sister is very moving: if the patient progresses well he will move on but if he dies, the nurse will share the family's loss and sadness

been accomplished it was clear that cyclosporin represented a major advance in clinical organ grafting. Many of the sceptics who had been sitting on the fence criticising the procedure now wanted to join the bandwagon and start organ transplantation themselves. The directors of Sandoz were amazed to find that the introduction of this drug caused a whole new branch of surgery to be developed worldwide, with cyclosporin as the major immunosuppressor for grafting the kidney, liver, heart and lung, and pancreas. (For reasons that were not clear, the intestine remained a stumbling block: rejection could not be controlled here even with cyclosporin. Nor could we transplant skin.)

A Miraculous Transformation

In 1984, Jane Bearstead, in her late twenties and a long-standing diabetic requiring insulin, was admitted with kidney failure. This was not the usual diabetic kidney damage but a glomerolonephritis not normally associated with diabetes. Nevertheless she elected to have a kidney and pancreas transplant. The operation was reasonably straightforward and she rapidly made a good recovery.

As a diabetic she had had difficulties controlling her blood sugar, having to take varying doses of insulin every day and follow a strict diet. Added to this were the constraints of kidney failure, feeling ill with anaemia, and needing kidney dialysis two or three times a week for six hours at a time. Her quality of life had been dreadful. To be cured of her diabetes and kidney failure in one operative procedure was an almost miraculous transformation. The two organs each had their own risk of surgical complications – the pancreas has a particular tendency to leak the powerful digestive juice that it produces. Jane needed to take daily immunosuppressive medicines but this was less of a burden than insulin and dietary control of diabetes, and the cure of her diabetes made her life much easier.

Jane returned home and, two years later, had her first baby. She was able to resume horse-riding and showjumping. She had a second baby two years later and now, sixteen years after transplantation, she is in good health, cured of her diabetes, and has a well-functioning kidney transplant.

The Mysterious Case of FK506

The saga of new discoveries in immunosuppression continued in the 1980s, with the mysteriously named FK506. At a meeting in Minnesota in 1982 I was chatting with some colleagues when a Japanese surgeon Takenori Ochiai, who had worked for a brief period with me and also with Thomas Starzl in Pittsburgh, approached in a conspiratorial way and said, *sotto voce*, 'I have a new drug a hundred times better than cyclosporin.' This sounded like rather more than a modest claim, and I asked him about the compound. He told me it was top secret, but divulged a few facts. His experiments had been done mainly with rats, and they certainly sounded impressive. I asked him if we could obtain some of the compound to carry out studies in other models and he said he would ask.

Not long afterwards I was visiting Japan and, after a number of communications with the Japanese pharmaceutical company, Fujisawa, I was told that it might be possible for me to do some experiments. Would I meet two representatives of the company in the lobby of the hotel? I appeared, casually dressed, and two very serious men approached me in perfectly tailored, identical grey suits. They bowed solemnly and started telling me about FK506, how it had been discovered in their laboratories, the tests they had done in tissue culture, and then Ochiai's experiments. I asked them if they could let me see the formula for FK506. They looked startled and exchanged glances. Then one of them, holding a book of data, flipped it open and, before my eyes could focus on the formula, he had closed it again, saying it was top secret.

Since I am not a chemist, the formula did not mean much to me, and it wouldn't have made a lot of difference if I had spent some time looking at this secret symbol. The outcome of the meeting was, however, satisfactory, and I was given an adequate experimental amount of the drug. We were able to repeat Ochiai's results in rats. But to say that it was a hundred times better than cyclosporin might give the wrong impression. It was effective in a much smaller amount, but the toxicity relating to the efficacy, the so-called 'therapeutic index', was not much different from cyclosporin's. When we tried the compound in large animals, however, it was exceedingly toxic and produced severe damage to small blood vessels all over the body. I felt, wrongly, that FK506 could not be used in man, but nevertheless I was extremely impressed by how effective such small amounts of this compound (a macrolide related to the antibiotic erythromycin) were in preventing rejection. It obviously had highly selective effects on the lymphocytes (white blood cells produced to fight infection).

The next chapter in the saga of FK506 came when Ochiai presented his data at the International Transplantation Society Meeting in Helsinki in August 1986. After his presentation I congratulated him, but also pointed out that the compound was toxic in large animals. Starzl was in the audience and, being very excited about these research results, shortly afterwards went to Japan for consultations with Fujisawa. Starzl than repeated the experiments that we had done and obtained results similar to ours, though he observed more effect and with a little less toxicity. His interpretation was entirely different and, as it turned out, correct, and he planned to try FK506 in man.

Studies in tissue culture showed that human lymphocytes were more sensitive to FK506 than those of animals. Starzl therefore started treating patients with a hundredth of the dose effective in monkeys. A veil of secrecy then descended on Pittsburgh for a few months until a meeting of the European Society of Organ Transplantation (ESOT) took place in Barcelona in 1985. ESOT is mainly a forum for European workers to exchange information and discuss new projects. Before the main meeting, however, there was a satellite symposium organised by Starzl through the Fujisawa company, which effectively hijacked that main meeting.

At this symposium, which went on all day until the late evening, Starzl's work with FK506, which had been extensive, was reported;

but, strangely, the drug did not seem to have any toxicity. Whenever the question of toxicity arose, the Pittsburgh team responded that they had seen hardly any untoward effects. FK506 was therefore hailed as the miracle drug from Pittsburgh. At the end of this symposium 1000 delegates left Barcelona – and never showed up at the ESOT meeting. This left the official meeting in disarray. For nearly three years no centre other than Pittsburgh could obtain FK506 to study it.

Eventually, when multi-centre randomised trials comparing FK506 with cyclosporin in liver transplantation were performed in North America and Europe, the results showed quite clearly that FK506 was a powerful immunosuppressant. If anything, it was slightly more effective for given toxicity than cyclosporin, but not different enough for there to be a statistical advantage as far as mortality and function of the transplanted organs were concerned. Despite the impression gained in Barcelona, the compound's toxicity was remarkably similar to cyclosporin's, including toxicity to the kidneys; it caused diabetes in some patients and neurological side-effects. So FK506, a compound with no molecular similarity at all to cyclosporin, appeared to be acting in a similar way. The puzzle was eventually solved: the mechanism, which is complicated, showed that, although FK506 and cyclosporin enter the lymphocyte by different routes, they both interfere with the same enzyme system that causes the cell to produce the stimulus for other cells to divide and attack the graft. The effect is rather like destroying the starter motor of a car, while leaving the engine intact but inactive.

The Easter Island Compound

I was so impressed with the effectiveness of FK506 in minute amounts that I wondered if there were any other macrolides of similar chemical composition which we might investigate for immunosuppressive properties. I had been spending a lot of time in discussion with colleagues and especially with the research group at Fisons Pharmaceuticals in England, who were at that time collaborating with the Fujisawa company. Although we looked at many different compounds and modifications of the original FK molecule, nothing seemed to be as good as FK506 itself.

In the literature, however, there was a report of a compound obtained from the soil on Easter Island, which was chemically very similar to FK506. The compound was called rapamycin, after the Easter Islanders' name for their home, Rapa Nui. The Ayerst Company in Canada had studied this material, which had been isolated by Suren Sehgal. Sehgal had found that it was a very powerful fungicide and it was hoped that the drug would be effective against fungal infections. Rapamycin also inhibited some tumours from growing. However, the experiments that Sehgal had performed on rats had disastrous results: the material caused the lymph nodes, thymus and spleen to shrivel up. Inevitably, this side-effect would make the compound unsuitable for treatment of humans with fungus infections or tumours.

The Ayerst Company was taken over by the huge American company Wyeth, and I wrote to them asking if we could have some rapamycin to study. Six months later I was told that I could proceed with experiments. We found rapamycin similar to FK506 in its effect on animals and we thought that its mode of action was probably the same. However, when the cell biology was investigated, it was shown to act in a completely different way, although it entered the cell through the same route as FK506.

This was, to us, an extraordinary and unexpected finding and probably very important, because when rapamycin was first used in humans, at about the same dose as FK506, it was found to be a powerful and effective immunosuppressant but with a pattern of toxicity quite different from that of cyclosporin and FK506. In particular, rapamycin did not cause damage to the kidneys and could apparently be combined with cyclosporin to produce a very effective treatment – more powerful, in fact, than the mere sum of two parts, a phenomenon known in pharmacology as synergy. This new agent, which has helped us understand how lymphocytes work, is currently going through its final trials and is due to be registered very soon.

Natural Tolerance

With every new immunosuppressive drug, we re-examine its possible use in producing general tolerance. In pigs and rats a transplanted liver can produce tolerance even without drugs. And even in man, a transplanted liver is less likely to be rejected than a kidney or heart – in fact, a significant number of patients have been able to stop using immunosuppressive drugs altogether.

Betty Baird is a particularly dramatic case in point. She had a new liver transplanted by Thomas Starzl when she was a baby in Denver. Ten years later she was well, but hated her appearance – the moon face and a tubby body that are a legacy of corticosteroids (part of the hated medical cocktail that she took to stop her transplanted liver from being rejected).

But Betty Baird wasn't going to take this lying down. One day she threw all her immunosuppressive drugs away and didn't tell anyone. She began to feel stronger and slimmed down, and she became attractive, like a normal youngster. Now, twenty-six years after her liver graft, she is the longest-surviving liver transplant patient in the world, and she has had no immunosuppression for the last fifteen years.

There are now ten patients who stopped all immunosuppression more than ten years ago and are well, but some patients with liver grafts stop immunosuppression, only to find that their bodies start to reject the graft. They then have to go back on to the drugs. This leads one to wonder what distinguishes Betty Baird and the lucky few others who have been able to jettison their drugs from other patients who can't survive without them. Obviously, Betty possesses natural immunosuppressive mechanisms, and it is the search for these that will dominate the next stage of transplantation biology.

Chapter Ten
The Media Circus

The media have always displayed a voracious appetite for all things medical, and especially for bizarre medical advances such as transplantation. Since the purpose of newspapers, television and radio is primarily to attract large and faithful audiences, for commercial reasons, a dramatic, emotional story – especially of a tragedy – is much preferred to a tale of successful progress without any disasters. It would be a foolish person who under-rated the power of the media and their ability to destroy somebody they don't like. Because of this power some journalists have an exaggerated view of their own importance. For example, my wife was once woken in the middle of the night by a reporter insistent on an immediate story on one of our liver transplants. She asked who it was and he said 'The *People*.' 'Which people?' she enquired, before realising that this was the name of a newspaper she didn't read. On another occasion, newspaper reporters came to our front door and demanded information, again about a liver transplant. Patsy explained that she didn't have this information and that they were pestering her in an unreasonable manner. They then became quite polite and said, 'Well, it doesn't matter, we'll make it up in any case.' (A notable exception is Fulton (Jock) Gillespie, of the *Cambridge Evening News*, who has always reported developments in transplantation sympathetically, responsibly and accurately, with compassion for patients.)

Television programme-makers are even more reluctant to take no for an answer. Researchers for topical programmes are prepared to seek individuals out wherever they are and whatever they are doing – they have even pursued me to the operating theatre by phone. I have had repeated prolonged discussions with people extremely ignorant of the whole subject who require an *ad hoc* seminar and often insist on an interview. On one occasion, at considerable inconvenience to my family, I complied with their wishes. After a long and uncomfortable journey to a distant studio, I was asked to wait and then an obsequious voice told me over the microphone that there had been a vote in Parliament which meant that they were going to cancel my part of the programme. I was assured that I would nevertheless receive a letter of apology and my expenses. It was no surprise that neither arrived and I eventually wrote to the chief of the programme. He replied with a polite, apologetic letter and told me that the expenses were on their way. Strangely enough, they still haven't arrived.

The Story of Ben Hardwick

Nevertheless, it is unhelpful to dwell too much on the negative aspects, since the mass media provide the main channel for informing the public of what is going on and explaining difficult concepts. It is just a shame that most programmes cater for such a short attention span that it is impossible to explain a complicated subject such as brain-stem death or the law on organ donation. Neither of these subjects can be fitted into a brief sound bite and so they tend to be passed over or diverted to a serious programme shown late at night to a minute audience. Doctors appearing on television need to be brave or stupid. They are out of their own environment and in the hands of clever professionals who have an easy time tripping them up as they wish and even making fools of them. Yet there have been important exceptions to this generally negative picture.

In 1984 we transplanted a little boy called Ben Hardwick, who soon became known to the whole of Britain as 'Little Ben'. Ben Hardwick came from an ordinary family and he was a very beautiful child with an extraordinarily engaging smile and laugh. But he was doomed to die from a liver disease. His bile ducts had failed to develop and he became increasingly jaundiced. The yellowness didn't hurt him, but the itching that accompanied it was hard for him to bear.

Ben was born on 6 December 1981 in Chessington and he was cared for at King's College Hospital in London. When he was two months old he had an operation to try and re-open the undeveloped bile ducts but sadly this was not successful. Mrs Hardwick wrote to me and asked if I could help Ben with a liver transplant that she had heard about from a friend in America. I wrote back explaining that we had not been offered any livers from child donors and at that time we did not have any other way of transplanting a large liver into a child. (Now, we can use the lobe of a liver, even from a parent, but in the 1980s we thought the only possibility was to obtain a liver of the right size.) Ben became very ill with an infection and, when he had recovered from this, Mrs Hardwick asked if she could bring Ben to see me, despite the minimal chance of obtaining a liver for him.

I explained to Mrs Hardwick the extreme sadness and sense of hopelessness that parents suffer when a child is killed in a road accident, and because of this, no doctors or nurses wish to intrude on their grief by asking if an organ can be removed to try and help someone else. My own personal view was that this thought of helping someone else can sometimes give a little comfort to bereaved parents, but this was not shared by most of my colleagues.

Mrs Hardwick said she would do anything and I said, 'Well, perhaps you can find a friendly television producer.' I knew the power of the media – and remembered the fact that a *Panorama* programme shown a few years previously had nearly stopped organ transplantation altogether by attempting to undermine the criteria of brain death using case illustrations from the United States that did not fulfil the criteria of brain death. This had been a disaster for the transplant world and many patients had died without receiving an organ as a result. Perhaps television could now restore the balance by helping Ben Hardwick.

A friend of Mrs Hardwick suggested that she contact *That's Life.* There was something about her entreaty that caught the attention and sympathy of Shaun Woodward and Esther Rantzen, and when they met Mrs Hardwick and Ben they were convinced that they should do everything in their power to try and obtain the gift of life for little Ben in the form of a new liver. On Sunday 15 January 1984 *That's Life* went out to an audience of thirteen million and portrayed Ben's plight with drama and compassion. This clearly aroused great sympathy among the viewing public.

On Monday 23 January a little boy with spina bifida died from associated brain damage and his parents gave permission for his liver to be used for transplantation. The liver had to be transported from another hospital, and was delayed due to snow, but the operation proceeded satisfactorily and was headline news for several days. All the publicity from this case was beneficial for the cause of transplantation. It helped increase organ donation of all kinds, and marked the beginning of transplantation of the liver for children in Europe.

Little Ben did extremely well to begin with, left hospital, and went home to his parents. But slowly, over the next few months, his liver function deteriorated, due to relentless rejection that did not respond to the immunosuppressive drugs. A few patients had been re-transplanted in the United Kingdom, but re-transplant operations have proved to be extremely dangerous due to the scars left by previous surgery, which makes it difficult and hazardous to remove the diseased liver. Thomas Starzl was visiting from Pittsburgh and nevertheless felt that the only chance for Ben was another liver transplant. So the desperate situation was explained to Mr and Mrs Hardwick, and they agreed to a second operation. By this time Ben had become jaundiced again and his condition was deteriorating, but he was still an extremely cheerful and bubbly child.

On Saturday 23 March 1985 the second transplant operation

was started. It began at ten o'clock at night and finished at six in the morning. It was extremely difficult and during the operation Ben's heart stopped but was re-started by an electric shock. An hour after the operation he had another cardiac arrest and this time there was no recovery. There was personal and public mourning for Ben but he remained a symbol of courage and the determination of a loving mother to leave no stone unturned. His story had touched the hearts of the public and changed attitudes towards organ donation. Esther Rantzen and Shaun Woodward deserve thanks from all the children who have subsequently been transplanted, including a namesake of Ben, Andrew Hardwick, who is now a healthy, strapping teenager, twelve years after his operation.

'That Will Do Nicely'

We had found that, although immunosuppression was needed for liver grafts, after a time some patients, like Betty Baird in the States, could stop the drug treatment without rejecting their grafts. Moreover, we knew that the liver would protect other organs from the same donor transplanted at the same time. We and others had had experience of combined liver and kidney transplantation with good results. In 1986 Dr Roger Williams referred Davina Thompson to me to be considered for liver grafting. This lady, with a non-malignant liver disease called primary biliary cirrhosis, was unusual because she had a rare and severe lung complication of this disease and required continuous oxygen administration from a mask. Needless to say, this caused consternation among the anaesthetists who said she was unfit for a hernia operation, let alone a liver graft!

I broke the bad news to Mrs Thompson, but she was a very determined lady and said we must do something for her. I explained to her that not only did she need a liver graft, but a heart and lungs as well, and that such an operation had never been done. Her response was 'That will do nicely.' So we approached our colleagues at Papworth Hospital, Cambridge, where the heart and lung transplant operations were performed, and the heart surgeon Mr John Wallwork agreed to collaborate in the proposed operation.

When a donor of suitable size and blood group became available we proceeded to remove the heart, lungs and liver from Mrs Thompson. Her circulation was maintained with a heart-lung machine. The empty thoracic cavity and absence of the liver below the diaphragm was a daunting sight, more reminiscent of a carcass in a butcher's shop than a surgical operation. The heart, as part of the heart-lung block, was not diseased and was therefore transplanted to another patient waiting for a heart graft (the so-called 'domino' heart transplant operation).

After some ten hours of work the new organs were perfused with blood and when the heart started to beat it was a beautiful sight for the surgical team. Mrs Thompson made an excellent recovery and was well, working full-time as a housewife, eleven years later. Her prophetic comments were realised – the new and untried operation did do nicely. Sadly, her heart and lungs were attacked by chronic rejection and she died peacefully twelve years after her operation.

When Mrs Thompson returned to Papworth Hospital for a follow-up, ten years after the operation, she was in excellent health and we organised a celebration party and held a press conference. However, interest from the media was minimal and the subject scarcely merited a mention in any of the national newspapers.

The Early Days of Heart Transplantation

In the eyes of the media, the drama of the operation seems to be more important than the long-term well-being of the patient, which is what transplantation is really about. This point has never been more forcefully illustrated than by the almost unbelievable razzmatazz that followed the first heart transplant in the world, performed in December 1967 in Cape Town by Dr Christiaan

Barnard. The event was covered by the media with the sort of enthusiasm normally reserved for the outbreak of a major war and had an extraordinary impact on cardiac surgeons worldwide. Since any cardiac surgeon can technically transplant a heart, there were few major heart centres where transplants were not attempted. The surgical results were usually satisfactory but most of the cardiac surgeons had no experience of transplantation immunology or immunosuppression and the infrastructure needed to prevent or control destructive rejection. Virtually all these poor patients therefore perished, having satisfied the macho aspirations of their surgeons. This series of failures had an extremely bad effect on the image of transplantation and resulted in a self-imposed moratorium on heart transplantation, except in a few centres where the procedure could be done with the appropriate infrastructure.

Dr Norman Shumway at Stanford University, California, had been a pioneer of experimental heart transplantation, working with Dr Richard Lower who later went to Richmond, Virginia. These two surgical scientists had demonstrated a satisfactory technique for heart transplantation: showing how to cool and preserve the organ so that it would function as a life-sustaining graft immediately; and how to use the chemical immunosuppression then available for kidney transplantation in patients receiving heart grafts. Dr Shumway's unit in Stanford University Medical Center thus became the foremost heart transplantation unit in the world. When cyclosporin became available in 1981 Dr Bruce Reitz, working in Dr Shumway's department, showed that this drug could prevent the rejection of combined heart-lung grafts in monkeys and then in man. This was the first successful grafting of lungs with good results.

Sadly, in 1980 the cardiac surgeons at Papworth in Cambridge were initially not prepared to use cyclosporin, even though we had shown its superiority over previous immunosuppressive drugs in both kidney and liver grafts. When they started their heart transplant programme, despite long discussions, they refused to depart from the orthodox (azathioprine and steroids), although they later changed to cyclosporin with enthusiasm. This is an interesting phenomenon that I have encountered repeatedly – that when a new treatment is first introduced there is always resistance to it. Once it has been accepted, there is similar resistance to it being superseded by a new and superior method proven in the laboratory or even in the clinic in another setting. Surgeons, like most people, are naturally very conservative animals.

The Tragic Case of Laura Davies

When considering the role of the media in transplantation the case of the toddler Laura Davies immediately springs to mind. Laura suffered from congenital liver and bowel disease, and in 1992 she was referred to me for an opinion. She came to Addenbrooke's with her parents and well-wishers from her home town of Manchester, all wearing special Laura Davies Support Club T-shirts. Sadly, this case became a media circus, as it was a recurring story in newspapers, radio and TV programmes. In the glare of all the publicity it was difficult to make a balanced assessment and give a useful opinion.

I explained that a liver and bowel transplant was the only treatment that could help little Laura. I was then forced to give a press conference and found my audience quite hostile. There was a strong desire to send the child to Pittsburgh where Dr Starzl and his team had carried out several pioneering multiple organ grafts. I concurred that this would be the best place for her to have the operation because of their unique experience.

In the event, the King of Saudi Arabia paid for Laura to go to Pittsburgh. However, after the liver and bowel operation, there were complications and she underwent a re-transplant, this time with six organs. Her condition deteriorated and sadly she died. Her coffin was carried through the streets of Manchester on a black hearse drawn by horses.

Laura's case raised a number of difficult questions. Is there a limit to what can or should be done technically? If the patient has already suffered grievously and disaster strikes, should even riskier procedures be attempted, with an ever-diminishing chance of success? Dr Tsakis, Laura's surgeon, said in retrospect that the second operation should not have been attempted, but it is easy to be wise after the event. Success would have produced a different conclusion.

The First Successful Six-Organ Transplant

Not long after Laura's death we were referred a young man, Stephen Hyatt, with a benign tumour that was strangulating the blood vessels supplying his abdominal organs. A victim of Gardner's syndrome, he had already suffered greatly. His duodenum, pancreas and most of his bowel had been removed; he required continuous morphia to control his pain and he was being fed intravenously. He wanted something done but we did not know if a transplant operation was possible. We said we would try and help him.

A patient of the right blood group and size, victim of a road traffic accident, developed brain-stem destruction. The family wanted any organs that could be used to be transplanted and on 15 March 1994 three surgeons, Peter Friend, Neville Jamieson and I, worked for more than twelve hours.

First the diseased abdominal organs (liver, stomach, pancreas, kidney, duodenum and small bowel) were removed, leaving the abdomen empty. Then the donor organs were inserted *en bloc* and they fitted into place in their new environment remarkably well. The surgeons had rest periods during the twelve-hour procedure, but one theatre sister, Celia Chan – as you may recall, a member of our team on the trip to China – worked the whole time. The patient's condition during the operation was precarious, and his survival was largely due to the brilliant skills of the anaesthetists and their technical team. The after-care was also critical.

On the ward round each day there would be a large gathering around Mr Hyatt's bed – a surgeon, hepatologist, gastroenterologist, renal physician and an endocrinologist. He managed to cope with all these doctors but for nearly three months he was miserable, as his new stomach did not work and he could not eat. Eventually the stomach woke from its slumber and for the first time Mr Hyatt smiled.

On the day of his discharge, the hospital chief executive, John Ashbourne, who had been amazingly supportive of our new endeavours, gave a champagne party and the press were informed that we had carried out the first successful six-organ transplant in the world. I had a strange *déjà vu* when another major gathering of the same newspaper, radio and TV reporters wanted to know all about the operation. I was then asked why Laura Davies had not been transplanted in Addenbrooke's. Some memories seem to be very short. I reminded them of the adversarial reception they had given me on this subject only a few months before.

Mr Hyatt is now well after five years, eating a little too much, and living a normal life with his wife and two small children. At no time has there been any suspicion of rejection in any of his six organs. I believe this to be due to the paternalistic protection of the liver and the overwhelming dose of donor antigen from such a large volume of tissue in the six grafted organs.

Dangerous Enthusiasm for Sport?

Later in 1994 I met Philip Jones who, in common with his two identical triplets, had a passion for football. When Philip was in his thirties, he broke his leg on the football field and was brought into hospital. There he developed terrible pain in the abdomen and was extremely ill. Surgeons operated on him and found that his small bowel was entirely dead, apart from the first few inches. While removing the entire bowel, they found a blood clot in the vein draining the bowel which had caused the catastrophe but they were unable to find any clotting abnormalities. Since Philip was one of identical triplets, he was sent to me as a candidate for transplantation, using a portion of bowel from one of his brothers.

I was worried that we did not know enough about intestinal transplants at that time to proceed in removing a substantial part of the bowel of a healthy person. I therefore consulted my colleague, Sir Miles Irvine in Manchester, who felt it would be reasonable to try feeding Philip through a vein, but he didn't do well with this. He became depressed and lost weight, his marriage broke up and he could not work. He came back to see me, wondering if we would reconsider a bowel transplant.

One of Philip's brothers was studied to make sure he would be a suitable donor and then we fixed a date for the operation. But both brothers declined to go ahead with the operation on that date because it was in the middle of the football season! Sadly, when the football season was over, the brother who had offered to give a portion of his bowel died.

A year later, the other brother, Peter, offered to give a portion of his bowel. We went through a great deal of soul-searching as to whether or not to go ahead, because by this time we had found that there was a mild clotting defect in the family which was presumably present in all three identical triplets. But the blood-clotting experts we consulted felt that the risk to donor and recipient would be minimal if we thinned the blood with anti-clotting drugs at the time of the operation and shortly afterwards. We therefore went ahead with the surgery.

Some 5 feet of Peter's small bowel were removed and the remaining bowel joined together again. Meanwhile the donor portion of bowel was cooled, but the vessels were not long enough to join so we had to take a small piece of vein from Philip's leg to make 'jump' grafts so that the transplanted bowel would have a good blood supply. Both the triplets recovered well and, since they were identical, no immunosuppressive drugs had to be given.

This was the first case so treated. (In America bowel had been transplanted between a pair of identical twins, but the doctors had given immunosuppressive drugs.) It is now more than two years since Philip and Peter's operation. They are both well and fully rehabilitated, with normal bowel function. They demonstrate to us very clearly how marvellous transplantation would be if we did not have to deal with the problem of rejection.

Another extraordinary case involving sport had occurred in the mid-1980s. Two girls in Germany were playing squash when one tumbled into the other, falling on top of her partner, who felt a terrible pain in her upper abdomen, where a knee had inadvertently dug into her belly. She was obviously very ill and was taken to the local hospital, where surgeons operated on her and found a rupture of the liver, involving both sides.

They tried to patch it up but the bleeding continued. They summoned Dr Ringe, a liver transplant surgeon from Hanover, who came with a team and found that the bleeding could not be stopped. The only way to save the girl's life was to remove the liver and divert the blood from the intestine to the main vein. This they did. A patient without a liver cannot live very long. After twenty-four hours of the most intensive treatment, trying to reproduce the liver's numerous vital functions, the efforts of even the most determined, skilful and well-informed doctors fail, and patients die.

Therefore, the victim of the squash injury needed a liver transplant, and, miraculously, a suitable liver was found after about seventeen hours. She started to do well but then rejection set in and she required a second transplant. The result was good and now, four years later, she is well. But who would imagine that a completely healthy person, after a minor tumble on a squash court, would end up without a liver and then eventually survive two liver transplants? Usually the most serious injuries on a squash court are to the eyes, head or joints – this liver injury must be unique.

To return to the subject of the media, it would be enormously helpful if reporters and programme-makers occasionally felt it appropriate to present transplantation in an unsensational, factual manner, explaining what we know, what has been done, where we still fail and what needs to be achieved in the future. The public would then understand that we scientists don't know everything; indeed, that we are still very ignorant of some of the fundamental aspects of transplantation immunology. We are also bedevilled by ethical dilemmas that previously didn't exist, and we need help in resolving the morally disturbing choices that confront us as a result of the success of organ transplantation.

Chapter Eleven
Home and Abroad

For someone interested in medical science, there can be few more agreeable places than Cambridge. An expert is close at hand in virtually every speciality and sub-speciality of science and the arts, the air is clear, and East Anglia is the driest part of the United Kingdom. We have an excellent train service to London, with a train every thirty minutes, making it easily possible to attend meetings and social functions and return to Cambridge on the same day. Having lived much of my early life in London, I still have an affection for that great city but Cambridge is an easier place in which to live and is sufficiently near for the attractions of London to be well within reach.

College Life

Like Oxford, the University of Cambridge is an arrogant institution, reluctant to acknowledge that distinction could occur in lesser institutions. These two old universities are centres of excellence but not humility and, although the majority of the Faculty at Cambridge are leaders in their field, there are also inevitably some lame ducks who seemed promising when they were young but have contributed little or nothing to their chosen subjects since. These are the people who tend to dominate the committees in the so-called democratic institutions that run the university because those doing important research do not have time to be involved in such activities. The result is an oligarchy of bureaucrats, resisting change from any direction but often being proved right in the long run in their reluctance to accept trendy innovations. The university originally evolved as a federation of individual colleges, each with its own governing body. But, as the technological aspects of university departments have become more and more expensive, central government funding has become necessary and, with it, a measure of government control. In theory the colleges are still self-governing and some are extremely wealthy, which permits independent action. Thus, under the stewardship of Dr John Bradfield as bursar, the fabulously rich Trinity College has not only helped poorer colleges but has also developed a large, mainly scientific, industrial site, the Cambridge Science Park. Many of the companies on this site work closely with the university.

Partnership between academia and industry is an interesting worldwide development. In the past, most distinguished universities would only accept money, grants and scholarships from industry or rich benefactors on condition that the university had the final say in how the money would be spent. In the last ten years, however, research funding from the government and major independent charitable trusts has diminished, and some research projects cannot be established without extra funds. Industry is now the only source of the huge amounts of money needed for some areas of research. Unfortunately, however ethical these commercial sponsors try to be, it is impossible for them to avoid influencing the expensive research projects they fund.

Academics who collaborate with industry are therefore serving two masters, the university and the industrial concern, and some may have a third master or mistress: their own personal gain. The combination of these three elements can make it tempting to depart from research stimulated by curiosity and the medical aim of improving the lot of suffering humanity. How we are to handle these temptations in the future I don't know; some kind of compromise will be necessary.

When it comes to clinical practice in hospital there are similar temptations – indulging in private practice in surgical specialities can increase income between two- and ten-fold. The more private practice the doctor does, the less time he can spend caring for the sick in the National Health Service (which is usually his primary job, at least on paper). The more money he gets, the more he seems to want: a 2-litre car must be upgraded to a 3-litre, and then to a 6-litre. Then one car is not enough, there must be two, and so on. The story is repeated with houses, yachts and luxury commodities of all kinds. There is very little control but fortunately there is much less abuse of the system than one might fear.

Trinity Hall

My college, Trinity Hall, is one of the oldest colleges (they were all called 'Hall' or 'House') in Cambridge. Founded in 1350, primarily for the study of canon and civil law, Trinity Hall still has a predominance of lawyers. Ten recent High Court judges in the United Kingdom had all been students at Trinity Hall. The college has 300 undergraduates and 100 graduate students in all faculties.

In the sixteenth century Henry VIII constructed several wonderful palaces, and he decided to build and endow the most splendid college yet in Cambridge. The teachers in Cambridge (who were all clerics) were delighted. But when the king said he would call his college Trinity, the fact that there was already a college dedicated to the Holy Trinity – Trinity Hall, next door to the proposed site – was tactfully pointed out. However, Henry VIII was not a man to be trifled with. Having noted, without much joy, the existence of Trinity Hall, he still persisted with the name of Trinity for his new and magnificent edifice. And so it is that every day letters come to one institution that are meant to be sent to the other, and people turn up in splendid evening clothes for dinners and parties at the wrong place and they are rapidly despatched to the college next door. One night the head porter at Trinity phoned his opposite number at Trinity Hall to complain of the noise our students were making. 'I am sorry,' said our head porter, 'but you should not have built so close!'

I find it difficult to explain this anomaly to visitors. Time and again, when they have been to dine with me in Trinity Hall, when I meet them again they say how much they enjoyed dining in Trinity. Of course if they had dined in Trinity they would know the difference because at Trinity Hall we have a magnificent kitchen which is the pride and joy of the Fellows and looked upon with envy by other colleges. We have a tradition of outstanding chefs who produce the most wonderful food, not necessarily elaborate but of a quality that would be difficult to obtain in the fanciest and most expensive restaurants.

Shortly after I was appointed a Fellow there were some complaints that the food was not sufficiently interesting. I was therefore appointed the first 'High Table Steward', an unpaid post which is my favourite college duty. I lunch once a week with the chef, the wine steward and bursar, and each week we invite one or two of the Fellows in rotation to find out what they would like to eat, hear any criticisms, and look at any special recipes that they would like tried out.

The college is small – there are now forty Fellows but there were under twenty when I was first elected. This permits friendship between Fellows and their wives or husbands so that if somebody is in trouble, others can rally round and help, like a family. It is interesting that the friendly attitude in Trinity Hall seems to be infectious. When a new Fellow, with a reputation for being difficult or prickly, is elected, it is surprising how quickly he seems to become civilised. Also, those who arrive declaring a total lack of interest in food are soon complaining if there is too much salt in the soup or the steak is over-cooked.

I regard my membership of Trinity Hall as a special privilege and I am grateful to the college for taking me in. In Oxford each professorial Chair is linked to a college but in Cambridge there is a quota of professors for each college, and a college under quota can offer a fellowship to a new professor but is not obliged to. Likewise, the new professor can accept an offer but, again, is under no obligation. Being a London graduate myself, I did not know very much about the Cambridge college system and, when offered a fellowship at Trinity Hall, I accepted without hesitation, although I was perhaps influenced by the fact that they had invited me to dinner, which as usual was excellent.

We were one of the first Cambridge colleges to admit women and I personally voted against this move. I thought it would change the ethos and atmosphere of the college but I was completely wrong. The main changes after admitting women were that the academic standards improved, and rowing became better than it had been for many years. The other change was that undergraduates tended to look inwards to the college rather than outwards to other activities in the university. This has narrowed the horizons of some undergraduates but otherwise the women Fellows, graduates and undergraduates have enhanced the academic standing of the institution.

Trinity Hall has been, for me, an important part of living and working in Cambridge. My four daughters were married in the college: in each case they enjoyed a superb wedding feast in the beautiful gardens, and left the celebrations by punt – with plenty of champagne. I have also played tennis and squash for the college for many years. An old academic and sporting friend is Peter Morris, who was appointed to the Chair of Surgery in Oxford in 1974, where he rapidly created an internationally famous surgical division excelling particularly in kidney transplantation. For many years we held a competition between our surgical departments in tennis in summer and squash in winter, preceded by an academic research meeting and followed by a party. These meetings were valuable academically but also forged friendships between the departments so that we were able to work together in science, rather than compete.

Dinner with Mrs Marcos

During the 1980s I had had several distinguished Filipino doctors work in my department, and in 1986 I was invited by Dr Ike Ona, now head of transplant surgery in Manila, to address the Philippines Kidney Society on kidney transplantation. As usual in the Philippines, the hospitality was warm and generous. The meeting was attended by doctors specialising in kidney disease and surgeons interested in transplantation, and after my talk Dr Ona and his friends invited me to a very simple beach-side restaurant where they served wonderful fresh fish. We dressed in casual clothes and drove out of Manila to a beautiful location. The sun was setting, and we had just reached the coffee stage of an enjoyable and friendly meal, when the patron appeared looking somewhat worried and asking Dr Ona to answer a telephone call.

Dr Ona came back, looking even more worried. 'It is Mrs Marcos, the First Lady, on the telephone. She is the patron of the Kidney Society and was sorry to have missed your lecture but would like us to go for dinner this evening.' I said that was very kind of her but, since we had already had dinner, perhaps we could explain this to her and thank her for her invitation. My response caused the silence that had already descended on the assembled company to change into an eerie, tomb-like stillness. Dr Ona slowly asked me a simple question – 'You do wish to leave the Philippines tomorrow morning, don't you, Roy?' The significance of his question did not escape me. I nodded. 'Shall I tell the First Lady that we will be delighted to join her for dinner?' I nodded again.

When the phone was down I protested gently that my stomach was full and that I was wearing a T-shirt and jeans. There was no time to change properly: I was lent a shirt and bundled into a car and we drove to an elegant French restaurant, allegedly owned by Mrs Marcos. Inside were thin, grim-looking men in dark suits, with guns bulging in their trouser pockets. After we had waited for some time (which thankfully permitted our stomachs to empty a little), Mrs Marcos appeared in a beautiful, blue, flowing Paris gown and I was seated on her right. I knew that her husband had had a kidney transplant and she started asking me questions about kidney transplantation but she did not seem interested in the answers during the elegant and, fortunately, *nouvelle cuisine* meal which was served very slowly. Instead the First Lady delivered a monologue lasting more than an hour and focusing on the important people she knew: Colonel Gaddafi, who obviously had been very friendly with her, which had helped with oil concessions; and Mr Andropov, who was apparently a charming man with a delightful sense of humour, who held Mrs Marcos in great esteem (rather than the sinister head of the KGB portrayed by the Western media).

I noticed that my Filipino friends were very reluctant to say anything unless it was dragged out of them and then usually replied with bland statements that could not be construed as critical in any way. I was less inhibited and some of my replies caused my Filipino friends to frown and I sensed that some of the dark thin men had put their hands in their trouser pockets. However, it all ended in a friendly manner with photographs, and the next day I caught my plane from Manila Airport without incident.

When I got home an unidentified caller from the Foreign Office asked if I had performed a kidney transplant on President Marcos. I explained that I had not even met the president. The caller didn't seem to believe this but did not pursue his enquiries any further. MI5 must have been following events, but from too far away to get their facts right!

The King and I

In the mid-1990s my ex-Cambridge Fellows in Thailand were organising a meeting in Bangkok and asked me to participate. King Bhumibol Adulyades, Honorary Fellow of the Royal College of Surgeons of England, had been on the throne for fifty years and the Royal College wished to congratulate him and give him their condolences for the loss of his mother who had died some months before. Since I was visiting Taiwan, the College Secretary, Roger Duffet, asked if I would deliver an illuminated congratulatory parchment and place a wreath on the tomb of the Queen Mother. I had been a medical student a year ahead of the Queen of Thailand's brother, Dr Kitikara, at Guy's. I had also been present ten years previously, when the honorary fellowship had been conferred on the King.

We were picked up (Patsy dressed in black and me with a black armband) by Dr Prasit Watanapa from Siriraj Hospital in a hospital car and conveyed to the Royal Residential Palace. Here, we met other officials of the Royal College of Surgeons of Thailand and were ushered into a huge waiting room, with beautiful purple and magenta orchids, large paintings of royalty, and two faded sepia photos of members of the Thai royal family.

More surgeons arrived, until there were eight of us, including the President of the Royal College of Surgeons of Thailand, Professor Arun Pausawasdi, who is Dean and Professor of Surgery. We were given a rehearsal for our audience with the King by a senior uniformed court official. Professor Arun would lead us into the King's room, we would bow and I would step forward, followed by Patsy, and we would shake hands with the King and bow. I would present the parchment and say a few words. After a dialogue led by the King, he would stand up and shake hands, we would bow and retire. This all took place as planned, but we were rather surprised when the King launched into a discourse which lasted one-and-a-half hours.

The King explained that the Buddhist religion did not oppose organ donation, and we agreed that superstition was a major stumbling block and public education was the way forward. I hoped the king might help with this, since he is loved and revered by his people. He asked me what I thought of the Chinese use of organs from executed criminals – a very sensitive issue – and I explained the views of the Ethics Committee of the Transplantation Society. He agreed there were important moral questions to be considered, and wondered if the fear and extreme pain experienced by executed criminals might harm the physiology of their organs. The King explained that he was writing his own memoirs, entitled *Agoraphobia,* and took some delight in the fact that most people present did not know what the word meant.

By the end, the King had talked for one hour and thirty-five minutes (on subjects ranging from his problems with angina to the dangers of flooding in Bangkok). I ventured a few comments and anecdotes. No one else spoke. It was a strange experience. He then arose and shook hands with Patsy and me, and we departed. At the end of the interview I was repeatedly bitten on the hands by a very large mosquito that also seemed to have been attacking the King. I eventually crushed it on my hand and it left an obvious splodge of blood. I wondered whose blood it was . . .

We then drove off to the Grand Palace where there was a floodlit temple, with the Queen Mother's mausoleum and many people seated outside wearing black. After a monk had intoned a mournful dirge we went inside the temple. There were more people sitting down and four sentries with purple-plumed helmets and rifles reversed. Professor Arun and I each carried wreaths and placed them on stands. Mine had silver flowers with 'Royal College of Surgeons of England' written on it; Professor Arun's had coloured flowers and was rather grander.

The Global Perspective

While on a visit to India in 1992 I was met at Bombay airport by the son of a colleague; both father and son were called Dr Doctor. As the young surgeon drove me through the streets around the airport he said that the people living in the streets of Bombay were thought to number two million. Although they received sufficient food to prevent malnutrition, they had no proper sanitation and often had access only to contaminated water. They lived in shacks – whole families in a minute space. Not surprisingly, infant and maternal mortality were tragically common. When I visited the children's hospital the doctor in charge told me that every day young patients, particularly children, were admitted *in extremis,* dying of tuberculosis, as well as typhoid and other bowel infections.

On leaving Bombay I spent a few days in Cochin on the south-west coast of India, an ancient and beautiful city with a reputation for tolerance of all races and creeds going back to Roman times. Here, I had time to muse on the quest for organ transplants and the irrelevance of hi-tech medicine and surgery in the context of the squalor and degradation of humanity found in most large cities in the developing world. It seemed that the alarming rise in world population, consumption of irreplaceable natural resources, and the misery of humanity concentrated in slum dwellings were partly a consequence of scientific progress, particularly in hygiene. This had decreased infant mortality but given us no control over the huge increase in births. Children, often unwanted by their mothers, were being born into an environment of filth and hopelessness. I started to write down some of these thoughts and soon found myself drifting into a fast-running and unfamiliar stream incorporating elements of reproductive biology, demography, ecology, religion, politics and human nature. These writings ended up as my book *Too Many People.*

It is estimated that in the next fifty years the population of India will exceed that of China (which is currently 1.1 billion). As a result, two of the most prestigious scientific academies in the world, the Royal Society and the American National Academy of Sciences, have published a warning:

> World population is growing at the unprecedented rate of almost 100 million people every year, and human activities are producing major changes in the global environment. If current predictions of population growth prove accurate and patterns of human activity on the planet remain unchanged, science and technology may not be able to prevent either irreversible degradation of the environment or continued poverty for much of the world.

In this context, it is true that our efforts in organ transplantation are irrelevant, and some of the criticisms directed at us may be justified. It is medicine, together with the teaching and practice of hygiene, which is largely responsible for the imbalance between birth and death rates, leading to a population explosion that can only be curtailed in a humane manner by birth control. The alternative is famine, disease, destruction of the environment and, inevitably, even greater conflict and war.

Human nature has not changed since prehistoric times: our primary instincts have always been to eat, drink and multiply. But the ecological balance between humans and other animals, plants and the environment has been gravely disturbed by the application of science. Along with medicine, jet travel and industry, new killing machines and nuclear energy are responsible for upsetting the delicate equilibrium. Since the scientific method is so effective, I believe it is the only approach that has any chance of restoring the balance between man and the rest of the planet.

The increase in the world's population is a subject that rises and falls on the agendas of international meetings, but it has never been very prominent in the political strategies of democratic countries – where politicians seldom think further ahead than the next election. In authoritarian, non-democratic regimes population can be controlled, as has been demonstrated in China, but the methods used have created a whole new set of social problems. In China there is now an imbalance in the male/female ratio, as female children are less wanted than male children, and are often neglected at birth so that they do not survive. Now that the policy of one-child families has been in practice for more than twenty years, the Chinese authorities are having difficulty managing a generation of spoilt, over-indulged young men who cannot find wives.

Although I believe we could, through our natural resources and scientific knowledge, control our continuing rape of the earth, it seems very unlikely that we have the will to do so. I hope this pessimistic view will be proved wrong.

In the context of all this over-population and human misery, how can we justify expensive high-tech surgery and where do the limits lie in transplantation? The pattern of progress seems to resemble that in athletic performance: whenever there is complacency in achievement, a new record is established.

Chapter Twelve

The Art of Surgery

There have been close links between artists and doctors, especially surgeons, since the Renaissance. Both disciplines require the study of anatomy, and some of the greatest painters were also experts in anatomy and physiology (Leonardo da Vinci being the most celebrated example). Image-making has two purposes which can coincide. The first is a practical, diagrammatic role (as in map-making or drawing up plans for a building), and this applies very much to teaching anatomy and surgery. The second aspect, the aesthetic side of the visual arts, is more difficult to define but has been a feature of all human endeavour, going back to paintings done in French caves 30,000 years ago. In my book *Art, Surgery and Transplantation* I have suggested that image-making is part of a general cultural instinct present in all human beings, in the same way as language.

Such common cultural activities include music, dancing, singing, poetry, sculpture, painting and drawing. Presumably they confer a survival advantage in the hierarchical organisation of a tribe or a community, the establishment and practice of religion, the seeking out of a mate, the staking out of territory, the warning of danger, and the mobilisation of group effort in avoiding or defeating a common enemy. These cultural activities are not to be found in our nearest relatives, non-human primates, nor in fact in most mammals. But they are all well developed in birds, especially the song and dance of courtship and the display of birds of paradise and peacocks. But the best example of artistic performance in nature is that of the bower birds, some twenty separate species of which are found in northern Australia and New Guinea. The male constructs an archway, a bower, or some other edifice of twigs, and on occasion has even been known to decorate the twigs with coloured berry juice or charcoal. He usually arranges an arena in front of the bower in which he performs his dance, the arena itself being decorated with shells from beetles, feathers from birds of paradise, and brightly coloured objects sometimes taken from human dwellings. The purpose of the bower is solely to attract a mate. It is not a place for nesting, protection or refuge. The more elaborate and beautiful the bower, the more likely the male is to attract an appropriate mate.

In humans, cultural achievements are often judged according to fashion. Nevertheless there is a remarkable conformity of aesthetic taste when it comes to appreciating the beauty of the human face. A few years ago an interesting study was undertaken using computerised images of faces. The average of 1000 face shapes was considered moderately attractive but members of both sexes usually reached a concensus on the most beautiful modification when viewing faces of either sex whether the viewers or the faces were Caucasian or Japanese. Although the amount of fat on the body that is considered beautiful is a matter of fashion, the contour of the face is not. And, just as the shape of the rose is considered beautiful, so there is agreement on the most beautiful face, male or female.

As a child, I was fascinated by drawing and colouring, and particularly enjoyed creating images of animals, aeroplanes and boats. In both botany and zoology my interest centred on the structural elements, and in order to learn them it was necessary to produce anatomical drawings of plants and animals. The function of the parts did not make sense to me without a mechanistic view of their inter-relationships. However, I also enjoyed painting landscapes, flowers and animals from a non-anatomical point of view. So, from an early age, I was interested in both the diagrammatic and the aesthetic aspects. I was taught well at school by Francis Russell Flint, son of the famous, early twentieth-century painter of nudes, William Russell Flint. Russell Flint was an inspired teacher who encouraged pupils to fulfil their own potential without being straitjacketed into a particular style.

I have painted intermittently all my life, mainly on holidays for relaxation, and I was taught to use the long Chinese brush for flower painting in the Chinese style by a friend and surgical colleague, Professor Earl Lu in Singapore. I also went to watercolour courses given by Ron Ranson in the Wye Valley. By the 1970s my interest in painting, and the time I spent on it, were increasing.

The Painter and the Painted

In 1988 the distinguished Scottish painter John Bellany had a liver transplant in my department and he did sixty paintings of himself while he was in hospital for three weeks. The pictures filled his room and the corridors and they were powerful images of a heroic figure, often suffering at the hands of doctors and nurses, with an expression on his face rather like that of St Sebastian as depicted in medieval paintings. Bellany and I became friends and he gave me some lessons, especially on the use of colour, of which he is a master.

In one of his lessons I had to paint him and I realised that my depiction of a really sick man recovering from a huge operation was very different from his own self-image. It also occurred to me that transplantation was a subject nobody had ever painted before because it didn't exist (apart from the legends of St Cosmos and St Damian transplanting a leg in the Middle Ages). Moreover, I had models who were captive while in bed in hospital and they were often pleased to have the chance of sitting, so that they could talk to the surgeon about little things that he otherwise wouldn't have time for.

Painting Patients

Children after liver transplants are particularly strong images to paint. Their faces reflect the suffering they have experienced and also their lack of understanding of what it is all about. They tend to regard doctors and nurses as the cause of arbitrary pain which bears no relation to any improvement in their suffering. They often appear to have very large eyes with extremely long eyelashes, a result of their malnutrition. I find the sketching of children a particularly important part of my attempts at painting. It also gives me a chance to get to know the children – they smile and are no longer so frightened when I enter the room. Seeing me sitting down without a white coat, with a piece of paper and a pencil, the children immediately relax, understanding that this is going to be fun and won't hurt.

Romesa, for example, was a six-year-old Indian girl who had a prolonged recovery period after her transplant. She was very pleased to be drawn and was delighted to have a black and white photocopy of the sketch which she could keep and colour in. These versions of the pictures, coloured in by the children themselves, help me to understand some of their fears and their courage.

Tamara Rainey, a child from Belfast, underwent four liver transplants. I did two paintings of her in 1990. Although she rejected all her grafts, and suffered a great deal, she was full of life and a very popular patient in the children's ward. In the end her brave fight ceased and she died of rejection after the fourth transplant. My picture of her, painting at an easel, was given to the Childrens' Hospital in Belfast as a tribute to a wonderful patient.

In 1992 I painted a very brave young girl called Jenny Hall. The picture reproduced in this book shows her sitting up in bed, recovering from her third liver transplant, holding one of her cuddly toys. The toy is a universal symbol of childhood, yet she had experienced more suffering in her life than most adults ever will. This is a painting which has been exhibited in many countries, was bought by a German doctor and now hangs in a hospital in Germany.

The intensive care nurse plays a vital role in the recovery of transplant patients and I have tried to convey this in a number of paintings. For intensive care nurses working with transplant patients, the relationship can be very poignant: sometimes the patient is unconscious, unaware of the care he is receiving; if he improves, he leaves the intensive care ward; if his condition worsens and he dies, the nurse shares in the sadness and sense of loss experienced by his family.

Also in 1989 I did a portrait of a child who became the first in Europe to be treated with FK506, the drug produced by the Japanese company Fujisawa from a bacterium that they isolated. When the Japanese representative from Fujisawa came to Cambridge he saw the child who thanked him in a most delightful way. The little boy had received a liver transplant but developed graft rejection symptoms which did not improve when he was treated with corticosteroids and anti-lymphocyte serum. However, when he was given the FK506 his condition improved rapidly. The portrait shows the puffy face which is a side-effect of the steroids; in the background is a picture of Mount Fuji, signifying the Japanese connection.

A year later, in 1990, I painted a very cheerful and optimistic young boy who was about to go to university. He suffered from Wilson's Disease, had fallen into a coma and had to receive emergency surgery. I painted him while he was recovering from the operation – he needed a tracheotomy and mechanical ventilation. Sadly, he died a few weeks later, after developing a lung infection. The portrait shows him smiling bravely but looking very ill, and my wife and I were worried that his parents would be upset by it. However, they saw it as a tribute to their son's courage and they asked for a copy of it.

In the same year, I did a portrait of a young girl of eighteen, during her recovery from a liver transplant. She suffered from porphyria, which causes liver dysfunction and photosensitive skin lesions. For this reason we operated on her in dim light. Afterwards, during her convalescence, she was kept in a darkened room in order to reduce her discomfort. Her mother, who kept a constant vigil beside her also appears in the painting.

In 1992, while visiting Pittsburgh, I painted Brian, a very courageous man who was waiting for a liver transplant from a baboon. Dr Starzl felt that a further look at xenografting was justified now that we had more powerful anti-rejection drugs.

Brian said that he expected the operation to be successful, but, if it was not, he hoped that the doctors would gain valuable information that would help other patients in the future. He was keen that I should paint the colour of his eyes correctly – they were green. He had his operation shortly after I met him and initially did well, but he later developed severe rejection and increased drug treatment led to infection. He eventually died – some seventy days after the operation. It was a sad end to his hopes, and those of his family and doctors.

Eileen O'Shea

Eileen O'Shea, a young nurse, was a memorable patient who agreed to sit for me. In 1990 she had developed liver disease unrelated to alcohol. She had a liver transplant, which appeared to be doing satisfactorily. However, on the tenth day after her operation, I was doing my ward round when I found her collapsed and in shock. An x-ray of her chest showed what appeared to be lung in the position of the liver, under the diaphragm.

It dawned on us that she had a most dreadful and previously unreported condition – isolated gas gangrene of the liver. Since the liver was poisoning her, we removed it immediately. It is very difficult to survive for an hour without a liver but, with intense effort and round-the-clock monitoring, the anaesthetists were able to replace most of the factors that the liver makes, and purify the blood with an artificial kidney machine (as the kidneys had stopped functioning when the liver was removed). In the meantime we telephoned all our colleagues to see if anyone could help with a donor liver as an acute emergency.

There did not seem to be any possibility of a liver in Britain, so we phoned our colleagues in France and Germany, and Professor Pichlmayr in Hanover generously offered to send us a liver that his team were removing for one of their patients. The liver was flown into Cambridge and we transplanted it twenty-four hours after Eileen had had her first transplanted liver removed. This saved her life and she rapidly improved.

Her kidneys recovered function but, unfortunately, the liver from Germany was of the wrong red blood cell group and was rejected in two weeks. We then performed a third transplant and initially she seemed to be doing well with this, but slowly rejection set in. It appeared that Eileen O'Shea was what Americans have called a 'liver eater'. She had developed a powerful immunity against liver transplants.

I did a series of sketches of Eileen and one day she came to my house and sat for a portrait in oils. She looked thin and jaundiced, and while she was sitting for the painting she asked me if she could have a fourth liver transplant. Her courage and determination to live were extraordinary.

Having been through this major operation with dreadful disappointments on three occasions, she wished to have a fourth chance. I said that I would try and perform a fourth operation for her and when I asked if she would like her transplants represented in the painting as livers or roses, she predictably chose roses.

Shortly afterwards we transplanted her for the fourth time and this liver was not rejected by her and she is well eight years later. This is a tale of extreme heroism in a young girl who had a close encounter with death on four occasions.

Brad Delve

Two years later, in 1992, I met Brad Delve, a young, energetic metal-worker with a zest for life; but Brad had inherited Gardener's syndrome. This is a disease which produces polyps in the bowel which turn malignant, and fibrous non-malignant tumours which can cut off the blood supply to the bowel. It can cause terrible abdominal pain and sometimes requires an urgent operation to remove the dead bowel before it kills the patient.

Brad had his bowel removed and was kept alive by intravenous feeding. In order to get enough nourishment into a vein he needed to spend most of his life, when he was not working, taking nourishment. The quality of his life was dreadful but he still continued to work.

With the encouraging results obtained from bowel transplants in London, Ontario and Pittsburgh, we decided to look again at this difficult organ which has such a tendency to reject. Even a slight rejection in the bowel may breach the barrier between the intestine and the blood; bacteria in the intestine can then flood into the bloodstream and cause terrible septicaemia, which can prove fatal.

We decided to treat Brad with FK506, as it is better absorbed than cyclosporin and the Pittsburgh surgeons had achieved superior results with this drug. A youngster had been killed in a road traffic accident and the parents wished all organs to be used. We tested the blood group and it was compatible for Brad. The operation was straightforward and Brad recovered well. The continuity of the bowel was restored and he went home eating normally. The first question he asked me when he came out of intensive care was 'When are you going to paint my picture?'

Because of his operation, Brad lost his job, which caused him great anguish, since he had managed to work previously. Despite letters from myself and other doctors, we could not get him restored to his previous employment. Nevertheless Brad was always cheerful and optimistic and he did well for three years. Then the function of his bowel deteriorated and, despite continuing with full-dose anti-rejection drugs, chronic rejection set in and the bowel became useless. We were planning to do another bowel transplant, as this was Brad's wish, but sadly he developed blood sepsis and perished. He was a man of great courage.

In the past eight years I have painted patients (both adults and children), colleagues, doctors, nurses and scientists, the operations and the donors. I have also become more interested in trying to improve my general technique in life drawing. Indeed, art has now become a major part of my life. Some people ask me if it is therapeutic but I find it more of a challenge. It is rather like the biology of transplantation – in the sense that we will never understand the whole story. Likewise, my paintings and drawings always fall short of what I would like. I think it is the continuing challenge that I find most interesting in both surgery and art.

The American surgeon Rudolf Matas wrote, 'In spite of the triple coat of mail with which the surgeon must often encase his heart in order to accomplish his tasks successfully, he is, nevertheless, a man, a human, and as such is unavoidably and most painfully affected by suffering and death when those overtake the young, the gentle and the beautiful.'

That feeling of devastation comes to me almost inevitably regardless of the age, disposition or beauty of the patient who has come to me for help. I am often haunted by the hopeful, trusting faces of relatives and patients for whom I have not done enough, no matter how desperate the situation before the operation. My old chief Lord Brock once remarked, 'There is no question but that the sorrows and bitter moments in surgery can fade before the great and intense satisfaction that comes when a difficult problem has been brought safely to a happy conclusion.' For me, painting distils the very essence of what Lord Brock was getting at and I hope that in my work I testify to the witness of Rudolph Matas.

I have exhibited paintings, especially at transplant meetings, in order to try and show the human side of transplantation, encourage organ donation and increase public understanding of the process. Transplantation is not just a dramatic operation (as the media loves to portray it) but a serious attempt to restore a doomed person back to a normal life for a long period of time. The relationship between artists and doctors continues to the present day. The coming together of surgery and art has, for me, been tremendously satisfying, if sometimes frustrating and disappointing, and there is plenty of room for improvement in both areas. The challenge continues.

Chapter Thirteen
Successes and Shortcomings

In my forty years as a surgeon I have seen many desperately ill patients who have miraculously survived and some of their stories appear in this book. For example, I remember a lady who had two liver transplants and spent eight weeks with mechanical ventilation, unable to speak, with a tube in her windpipe. Every day she received encouragement from Dr Graeme Alexander who would whisper in her ear, 'Don't give up, you are going to get better.' Then there was an Israeli lady, similarly afflicted, whose loving husband came every day and played her Hebrew songs on a harmonica while she was unable to respond, also with a tube in her windpipe. But I have never witnessed anyone who showed more courage and determination, in the face of apparently overwhelming disease, pain and disappointment, and yet remained smiling, than Evan Steadman.

A very tall, white-haired man, aged sixty, first came to us with advanced cirrhosis and did well with a liver transplant for three years, but then the liver was rejected and he was given another transplant. This failed rapidly and he had a third liver graft. He became extremely ill and his body was racked by infection. His spleen was removed. After a few months he left hospital, only to return, looking like death, when he was found to have a cancerous growth in his pancreas. Despite the sepsis, the immunosuppressive drugs, the many operations and the disappointment of apparently getting better and then relapsing, he went through a huge cancer operation. And when his mouth was sufficiently free of tubes he managed a smile which has got bigger ever since.

Now, three years later, he is running a highly successful business, employing twenty-one people, and wants to do his best to help transplant patients of the future who are unlikely to suffer as grievously as he did. My colleagues and I were amazed and humbled by his indomitable spirit – he was a source of inspiration to us all.

The Good Samaritan

Brian Scott was another memorable patient. He had an amazing story to tell when he came to see me in 1997. He had been working on the production side for an English pop group in New York. One sultry evening in 1984 he'd been strolling along the sidewalk when he heard a commotion. An old lady carrying shopping bags was being set upon by three thieves who knocked her to the ground. One hooligan had his foot on her neck and the others were dragging her bag from her.

The streetwise New Yorkers who saw the incident just walked past, but Brian's sense of outrage triggered a reflex to try and help the defenceless victim. He chased the hoodlums but one of them lunged at him with a knife. In the course of the scuffle he noticed a sharp pain in his side. The thieves ran off and he comforted the terrified woman. He then felt something warm and wet on his body and realised his hand was covered in blood.

He was taken to the emergency department of St Vincent's Hospital and the stab wound was examined by the doctors who felt that there could be serious internal injuries and he needed an emergency exploratory operation. He woke up to find a surgical cut stretching the whole length of his belly and a blood transfusion pouring into a vein his arm. The New York Police Benevolent Society paid his medical bills.

At the time he did not realise, nor did the doctors, that the blood transfusion contained a potentially lethal virus, hepatitis C. It had been a mystery for many years that some patients were afflicted by severe liver disease without having any evidence of the two recognised viruses A or B. The liver doctors used to call this disease Non-A non-B hepatitis – a very awkward term. The mystery was partially resolved when hepatitis C was discovered. This virus can cause a slow and deadly cirrhosis, with a predisposition to tumour formation. Thirteen years after the blood transfusion, Brian became ill and developed symptoms of these complications.

The only effective treatment we could offer him was a liver transplant. I first met him the day before I was to perform the operation and he told me the story of his New York adventure. I could not imagine a more deserving recipient for a liver transplant and fortunately the operation went well. Like the Good Samaritan in the Bible, his charitable act was inspired by compassion for an innocent weaker person violated by cowardly thieves but he had suffered more grievously than the Samaritan.

I witnessed another charitable act in my department later that year. Alan Wildsmith, a man in his fifties who lived locally in Cambridge, had been on dialysis at Addenbrooke's for years. He had a stable family and a loving wife, Monica, who wished to give him a kidney.

She had heard that spouse-to-spouse kidney transplants did well, probably partly because the kidney is transplanted immediately without suffering damage due to preservation. Also, when a spouse gives a kidney, he or she is usually most anxious to make sure that the recipient takes his or her medicines conscientiously so that the kidney gift is not destroyed.

We explained all the hazards to the couple and Mrs Wildsmith was determined to go ahead. So we proceeded with the operation, which was straightforward, and both husband and wife recovered well and quickly, and are now living happy, normal lives. A tribute to marital bliss.

The National Health Service in the 1940s

I have worked in the National Health Service almost since its inception. Organ transplantation obviously takes place in the context of the NHS as a whole, and it is instructive to look at the evolution of Britain's health service, which involves all citizens to a greater or lesser extent and consumes a significant proportion of the gross national product. To understand the present (and future) state of the NHS, and the problems faced by today's health-care professionals, we need to start by looking at medicine in the past.

In 1947, when I was sixteen, the pattern of disease was very different from today. There were 20,000 deaths a year from tuberculosis and several of my contemporaries were undergoing treatment for that condition, spending months on cold balconies of the medical block at Guy's. We would attend ward rounds shivering, though the consultant was usually sensible enough to wear an overcoat. The poor patients seemed to take this treatment – imprisonment on a freezing balcony, their drinking water turned to ice – with remarkable equanimity and good humour. It was doubtful whether the regimen helped them, but it certainly limited cross-infection. If they improved they were sent to the Swiss mountains to convalesce.

Meanwhile, patients with chronic osteomyelitis lay in the orthopaedic and general surgical wards, their wounds pouring evil-smelling pus for weeks, months and occasionally for years. Acute poliomyelitis was common, and many of those who were not lethally affected required prolonged or even indefinite mechanical lung treatment at special hospitals such as the Nuffield Orthopaedic Centre in Oxford. There was no established cardiac surgery, although early pioneer work was underway, and organ transplantation had not been heard of. There were no counsellors, social workers or accountants, and administration was dealt with by a minimal office establishment headed by a senior consultant (the medical superintendent) whose word was law and whose judgement was generally wise.

The wards were run exceedingly efficiently by a ward sister who had supreme authority. The nurses' uniform, hair length and general manner were ordained by the matron's office and transgressions could lead to dismissal. The medical and surgical firm structure also followed a strict hierarchical system. I did three house jobs at Guy's, and in each case, as the most junior doctor on the firm, it was my duty to open the door of the Rolls-Royce when the consultant arrived. The registrar and senior registrar would lead the ward round and responsibility for any defects in the patient's notes, treatment or management would rapidly filter down to rest firmly and painfully on the poor houseman's shoulders.

Nevertheless there was a friendly atmosphere, most of us taking pride in trying to do the job well. And there was a certain satisfaction in sitting down with the consultant, sister, senior registrar and registrar to beautifully prepared cucumber sandwiches and Earl Grey tea. A houseman's annual pay was £250 and we had to stay in the hospital for the whole of each six-month period. We certainly couldn't leave the hospital when we were on call, although, when work in the ward was light, the consultant usually turned a blind eye to this rule. Often at the end of an emergency take period, there were noisy parties that would not now be tolerated.

The attitude of the hospital to patients was generous – poverty-stricken pensioners in the borough were often admitted at Christmas so that they could have roast turkey and enjoy the hospital festivities, subsidised by well-wishers. Decisions tended to be taken on common-sense grounds, with the benefit of inside knowledge from the sister and the almoner (who were the equivalent of today's social workers) without the jargon and the bureaucratic rules that now burden us. Patients with arthritis were doomed to stay in wheelchairs or their beds for the rest of their lives – there were no artificial joints; diabetics became blind early in the course of their disease; and elderly patients with pneumonia and children with cancer died. The hospital tried to make their final days as comfortable and pain-free as possible, administering generous doses of the Brompton Mixture (morphia, cocaine and brandy). Operation lists continued until all the patients had received treatment; last-minute cancellation was unheard of. Society was very different: expectations were low and patients were grateful for any treatment they received. Nurses were highly respected in the community and a Guy's nurse wearing her uniform and cape could walk safely anywhere in the borough, a rough area, because the local residents knew that the hospital and the nurses in particular were devoted to their care when they were ill.

The National Health Service Today

All this was true only fifty years ago. Yet the picture I have painted could almost be a century old, so extraordinary are the changes which have taken place. First, there has been a complete democratic levelling. Nurses and Sisters are on first-name terms. Sisters are frequently advised not to admonish juniors since the consequences may well be complaints to the hospital management and hours of wasted time, frustration and perhaps even anguish if the junior is exaggerating a perfectly justified telling-off. Junior doctors work in shifts and there is no longer any continuity of care. Patients are 'handed over' when the junior doctors have finished their prescribed hours; only the consultant retains overall responsibility.

The changes in medicine and surgery have also been enormous, as my own story has amply shown. Imaging techniques now give the surgeon a three-dimensional anatomical view of the patient's insides, rendering the skills of clinical diagnosis and localisation of disease (once so highly prized) redundant. The surgeon may be presented with the equivalent of a 'cut along the dotted line' instruction in a child's model-making kit. Many procedures can be dealt with using minimally invasive techniques. The radiologist and the physician have taken over several areas that were previously the domain of surgeons; complicated cardiac surgery is now routine, with the function of the heart and lungs safely provided by a machine during the operation. Arteries can be operated on, joints replaced, the retina and virtually all parts of the eye and the ear can be approached using micro-surgical techniques, and the flexible endoscope (a British-invented telescope that can look round corners in the stomach and bowel) has revolutionised much of surgery. Most of the vital organs can be transplanted successfully.

Patients' expectations are high and the present administration encourages them to complain when they are dissatisfied. When I first came to Cambridge grateful patients would often bring a pheasant or a bottle of wine after treatment; now a complaint is more likely. While negligence or inappropriate treatment should, of course, be identified and the injured person compensated, there is now a tendency for a small minority of patients to regard any untoward happening or unsatisfactory outcome as a failure of the hospital. Every week most consultants are therefore bombarded with trivial complaints – in Addenbrooke's they come in red despatch boxes. For example, one patient informed me that the nurses in the ward didn't like her (which I expect was a correct interpretation of their feelings) and that she was given cold toast – hardly matters for a surgeon. Even more ridiculously, it was recently reported that a patient treated for cancer had survived longer than predicted; he had therefore been granted legal aid to sue the doctors who had given him a gloomy prognosis.

Virtually all new treatments are expensive, and intensive care beds cost £1,300 a day. For this reason, there has been a tendency to move patients out of the hospital into the community, with fresh wounds and even drains still in place. Wards have been shut, leaving insufficient ordinary beds for patients, and there has been a drastic failure to provide sufficient intensive care facilities. Previously, extra beds were put up in corridors; now such an action would be condemned and considered a breach of health and safety regulations. Better to leave the sick patient to his own devices out of hospital, the thinking seems to be.

This situation is partly due to doctors, who naturally like to be big fish in small ponds and resist with great force and much shroud waving any attempt to rationalise critical care. The present system consists of small units which alternate between gross overwork (with staff leaving because of the stress) and underwork (with staff leaving due to boredom). The anaesthetists have become a very powerful lobby group and in our hospital cause many operations to be cancelled. This means that doctors, who are being paid high salaries, cannot fulfil their work allocation. And if they have nothing to do there is a natural tendency for many to work in the private sector, where operations are very seldom cancelled and they always receive a warm welcome. Consultant surgeons are paid for cancelled sessions and then paid extra for sessions at weekends to avoid the Health Trust being penalised for having long waiting lists.

This is all an intolerable waste. The new government has sensibly abolished the system of negotiation between providers and purchasers, in which the health authorities' highly paid accountants spent many happy hours playing a bargaining game with 'Monopoly' money – that is, health service funds. It is not surprising that the morale of workers at the coal face suffered, and many staff resigned because of the excessive bureaucracy and unhappy working conditions. Now the wards expel all but the dying at Christmas, there is no turkey to carve and little good cheer.

In general practice the situation is also unsatisfactory. Many fund-holders have been turned into bureaucrats, although they have not been trained for this role and most are not good at it. In recent years, when I have asked my students what they wish to do, few have said that they want to go into general practice, whereas previously that would have been the first choice for the majority. Inner-city general practice is particularly unpopular and can be dangerous, so there is a shortage of applicants for posts and therefore overwork and frustration for those left holding the fort. Many young doctors don't know what they want to do. They don't like the idea of NHS hospital practice either, and 20 per cent leave the health service within five years of qualifying.

Questions have recently been raised as to who should be treated, and in some hospitals smokers are not allowed to have arterial or cardiac surgery. In my unit nurses felt that alcoholic liver disease should not be an indication for liver transplantation but when I asked them what they felt about treatment of road traffic accident victims as a result of reckless driving or driving when drunk, they felt that that was different. They were not so sure when I asked them about treating a youth who was drunk and killed children waiting for a school bus. These are not straightforward questions for which there are simple answers.

How Can the System be Improved?

Assuming the picture I have painted is approximately correct, what can be done? It's no use simply blaming the government. No matter what type of health-care system we have, there will never be enough money to cover the spiralling costs of high-tech medicine and surgery, and this is a fact of life even in the richest countries. So is it possible to improve on the system we have at present?

Super-specialisation may be one way of significantly improving the situation. The arguments in favour of it are strong. To get really good results safely, one needs to have continuing experience and practice in a technique and, for this to happen, selected cases need to be sent to the appropriate specialist. In North America, for example, specialist surgeons are appointed to institutions solely to do keyhole surgery on the knee joint or the gall bladder or their practice is confined to repairing hernias or treating piles. And any patient coming to one of these doctors with a complaint which does not fit into their narrowly defined speciality must be referred to a more appropriate specialist. In Britain the increasing tendency to sue doctors, and the decisions of courts to award enormous damages for negligence, are persuading hospital managers to restrict the activities of specialists to their chosen field, and each speciality becomes further subdivided each year. Whether we like it or not, this trend towards specialised subdivisions of surgery and medicine is inevitable and will continue in the future.

It costs more than £200,000 to train a doctor. This generous investment by the tax-payer should be honoured by service in return. Ten years of work in the NHS would seem to be a reasonable requirement for medical graduates who have been financed by public money. If they wish to leave the NHS before ten years is up, then a proportion of the fees should be paid back to the Treasury. As many as 14 per cent of those admitted to medical school never complete their pre-registration year (in addition to the 20 per cent who leave within five years). This is a serious waste of money. A traditional medical training will still be needed for general practitioners and doctors practising emergency medicine and surgery, those working in isolated areas or in developing countries. Widely trained doctors will also be needed in every hospital undertaking highly specialised work. If, however, we look at the current state of medicine and surgery, and the way in which it is developing, it seems that a different form of training would be more appropriate for many specialist practitioners. Life is too short for all surgeons to obtain the appropriate 'trade union ticket' for each sub-speciality, and the expensive equipment required for many of the new techniques will probably not be available in small, isolated hospitals.

There is already a precedent in the heart/lung bypass work of perfusion technicians. Although they do not have formal medical training they have to take responsibility for the delicate technical management of the heart/lung machine and they need to react quickly should any malfunction develop. Special training for this new type of technological surgeon would lessen the burden on the tax-payer and would be appropriate for the work involved.

Widely trained general surgeons and physicians would still be needed to assess patients – for instance, to point out that cerebrovascular disease would make intervention in the knee irrelevant, or that diabetes needs to be controlled before the gall bladder is removed. But for the specialist of the future, an initial Bachelor of Science course in general anatomy, physiology and pathology would be a suitable start. Then, instead of clinical training in all branches of medicine, surgery, gynaecology and obstetrics, the next three years could be devoted to training in the speciality the student wishes to embrace – rather like the old apprenticeships in trade guilds. The universities would still need to have the traditional departments teaching anatomy, physiology and pathology for both the generalists and the super-specialists. The super-specialists should receive satisfactory remuneration for their responsible work with specialised techniques, but they should not be in a position, through their individual trade unions, to exploit the community with outrageous fees.

Audits could easily be achieved by storing video recordings of each operation in a computer. These could be played back to show if, when and exactly how mistakes had been made, and whether they were due to negligence or failure of equipment. With continuing experience in a narrow field, serious errors would be unusual. The situation would be similar to that of a highly trained air crew on a flight deck, each knowing their job thoroughly and reacting immediately to any sign of danger. The super-specialists are becoming rather like airline pilots who, after a short general training, are selected to manage one type of aircraft, say a Boeing 747. They are only allowed to fly a Boeing 747 and cannot transfer to another aircraft without lengthy retraining. Their licence to work as a 747 pilot depends on their clocking in a certain number of hours' flying a year.

Much of the work of super-specialist doctors would be very monotonous and repetitive. Oxbridge-type selection, requiring three As at A level, would therefore be inappropriate for somebody whose life would be spent, for example, operating within the confines of the knee joint. Likewise, someone with a wonderful brain but poor hand–eye co-ordination would be totally unsuitable. The universities will undoubtedly need to change their selection procedures to staff the brave new hospitals of the future with orifice and keyhole technologists, since these forms of surgery are definitely here to stay.

Registration and training of health-care workers need to fit the new pattern of medicine and surgery. This proposal will no doubt be violently resisted by the medical establishment (specialist associations, medical and nursing councils and the Royal Colleges). We need vocationally motivated people taking care of sick patients cheerfully, making sure their bodies are washed, and that they get food and drugs at the right time and especially pain relief. We also need general practitioners able to spot the really sick patients early and refer them to the right person. Most of the general practitioner's work involves relatively minor ailments. They should be helped by nurses who have been trained in a variety of special areas. These nurses could take blood pressure, give injections and prescribe simple medications. Other nurses might train to be operating theatre assistants, doing simple surgical procedures under supervision. Others would give anaesthetics, under supervision, as is the practice in the United States.

The specialist associations will probably throw up their hands in horror at these suggestions, particularly because it is well known that an intelligent nurse with special training could do most of the jobs that doctors do just as well and sometimes better.

A Typical Surgical Emergency

Throughout my surgical career I have always maintained a major interest in general surgery and especially surgery of the blood vessels. When I was a student, a ruptured artery was a death warrant. Nowadays more and more patients are saved, although the mortality rate is still high. Changes in this area of health-care over the past fifty years have been astounding. Every organ transplant requires joining of blood vessels, control of clotting, and, above all, prevention of bleeding. Working in a wide field of surgery, operating on different parts of the body, gives one an overview which is becoming more and more difficult to obtain as surgery becomes increasingly specialised and restrictive. As I have said, super-specialisation is inevitable but we will always need people who are capable of looking at the big picture.

I still do on-call emergency surgery and one of the most terrible common emergencies is a burst aneurysm in the abdomen. The main artery of the body, the aorta, passes through the back of the abdomen in front of the spine, giving vital branches to all structures on its way. A ruptured aneurysm is an extremely dramatic, and often rapidly fatal, complication of atherosclerosis. Usually blood vessels affected by this disease become obstructed by the hardening of the arteries and laying down of clot – rather like the furring of a kettle. When an aneurysm forms, the atherosclerosis causes a weakness in the wall of the blood vessel which begins to dilate like the inner tube of a weakened car tyre. The swollen artery may continue to enlarge very slowly for a number of years, or the swelling may progress quickly. In a thin person, a pulsating lump may be seen in the centre of the abdomen and it can be felt easily when a hand is laid on the belly. In a fat person, no abnormality may be felt or seen despite the presence of a large aneurysm. The fear is that the aneurysm will eventually rupture or 'blow out'. This may occur first as a small leak (contained by the membranes around the artery), or there may be a catastrophic loss of the whole circulation into the abdomen, resulting in immediate death.

Unfortunately, even relatively small aneurysms can rupture and they are very difficult to detect except with ultrasound scanning. For this reason, it has been suggested that everyone over the age of, say, sixty should be scanned once every two years, but this would be a huge and very expensive undertaking. If an aneurysm is detected, but it is not causing any symptoms, by far the best option is to remove it and replace the artery with a cloth tube. This operation has very good results and a low mortality.

A burst aneurysm may kill immediately but a leaking aneurysm may cause symptoms that permit the patient to be admitted to hospital. Then really urgent treatment is required to give a chance of recovery.

The organisation of the operating theatre and personnel for this crash-type of operation is well rehearsed in large teaching hospitals. But the patient may still undergo a terrifying ordeal before the merciful anaesthetic is administered. The operation for a burst aneurysm has a survival chance of between 20 and 50 per cent.

William Clarke was a not untypical case. He was enjoying his retirement after forty years working on the railways, first as a steam-engine driver and then as the driver of a diesel train. He had a little terraced house in Cambridge. His pride and joy was his small garden, which was the envy of his neighbours, many of whom also had beautifully maintained gardens. One October afternoon he was pruning his favourite roses when he suddenly experienced a severe stabbing pain in the lower part of his back. He thought it was his arthritis catching up with him again, but the pain became worse and he felt sick, and he realised that it was not the arthritis but something else.

When the pain became really dreadful, and terrifyingly persistent, his wife phoned for an ambulance and he soon arrived in Addenbrooke's Hospital. The on-call senior house officer immediately realised that something very serious had occurred. The site of the pain was unlike a coronary thrombosis and William Clarke's pale complexion, and the vague pulsation still apparent in the centre of his abdomen, told him that this was probably a case of a leaking aneurysm.

The senior surgical registrar was summoned urgently. He agreed the diagnosis, assessed Mr Clarke's general condition, and pronounced him otherwise remarkably fit for a man of seventy-seven. He gave Mr Clarke an injection of morphia for the pain, explained to him that he had a burst major blood vessel and required urgent surgery, alerted the operating theatre, and called for porters to bring Mr Clarke immediately to where a senior anaesthetist was waiting. He explained briefly to Mrs Clarke the nature of the condition and the desperate need for an operation which was often unsuccessful. She didn't understand all that was said to her, but she fully realised that the situation was grave.

A general anaesthetic causes a drop in blood pressure, and a patient with a burst aneurysm is usually already suffering from low blood pressure due to blood loss. On the other hand, too forceful a replacement of blood through a vein may raise the blood pressure and cause the bleeding to be more rapid and severe. The anaesthetist and his team therefore need to prepare the patient in the operating theatre rather than the anaesthetic room, so that the surgeon and theatre sister have all their equipment ready, the patient's abdomen cleaned, surgical drapes applied, and the knife ready to make an incision. Only then does the anaesthetist give a general anaesthetic, pass a tube into the airway and ventilate the patient.

Preceding the surgery, the patient, fully conscious and in dreadful pain (with some relief from morphia), is wheeled into the brightly lit operating theatre. There are many people there, none of whom he knows, and they have little time to extend human kindness as well as clinical efficiency. The main priority is to achieve a good surgical result. Inevitably, instructions are issued, voices are raised, and egos are bruised, as more senior or experienced people join the team. I think all this must seem like bedlam to the poor patient – a dreadful environment in which to start a journey into the unknown with a high risk of death either during the operation or from complications afterwards.

When the intravenous anaesthetic is administered and the unconscious intervenes, the team can proceed. The surgeon then makes an extraordinarily long cut, from the pelvis up to the chest. At this point, everything depends on whether the initial bleeding can be contained, and the active bleeding removed by two powerful suckers, so that the surgeon can see to get a clamp above and below the aneurysm. This may be extremely difficult as there is a danger of damaging the blood vessels to the kidney. The process of clamping the aorta may also result in tearing of the aneurysm and more bleeding. In theory the operation is a simple one. The artery is clamped above and below the blow-out, the blood clot is sucked out, and a cloth tube is sewn to the artery above and below the blow-out, which is thus excluded from the arterial tree. However, aneurysm patients often already suffer from atherosclerosis in their coronary arteries (the same hardening-of-the-arteries disease which caused the aneurysm), and heart failure is a common cause of death in the post-operative period. The kidneys may not function properly afterwards and artificial kidney treatment may be required. Lung infection is common.

In William Clarke's case, despite difficulty in getting the clamps on above and below the aneurysm, the clamps were applied, the bleeding stopped and an expensive Dacron tube was sewn to the artery above and below. (With skilled anaesthesia, the clamping and unclamping of the blood vessel can be tolerated by the heart.) The operation was completed in two-and-a-half hours. At the end of it Mr Clarke's condition was stable, the anaesthetist and surgeon were pleased, and he was taken to the intensive care ward.

He half woke up the next day to find that he could not speak and had a tube in his airway. He couldn't move and his arms had painful needles in them. A kind nurse hovered over him and there were intermittent visits from doctors, physiotherapists, radiographers, and his wife. The next day he was lucky: his breathing muscles were strong enough to cope on their own, the tube could be taken out of his airway, and he could speak again, although initially his voice was very hoarse, and his abdomen felt dreadfully painful. The doctors seemed happy that there was no more bleeding but the tube in his bladder was very uncomfortable and the whole procedure had been a nightmare from which he had not yet full awoken.

Two weeks later, when he was ready to go home, I asked him what he remembered of the time just before the operation. He said, very little except that he was in terrible pain, and it was a dreadful experience.

Mr Clarke was a lucky patient. Similar cases may be less fortunate and fail to survive the operation or may succumb to complications afterwards. Aneurysms appear to be becoming more common, perhaps because patients don't die from other diseases. Our hospital handles approximately 100 aneurysms a year. But managing them requires a staff of highly trained surgeons with sufficient experience of the condition and this is difficult to arrange in any hospital. Surgeons in training nowadays spend less time learning different techniques, and one should not be faced with a burst aneurysm as one's first experience of performing this operation solo. Clearly, we need more surgeons to cope with this disease, but how can a cash-strapped health service provide appropriate facilities for aneurysms, mostly for elderly people, when the waiting lists for simple operations are increasing all the time? The painful nettle of rationing will have to be grasped, although the very word causes shudders to run through politicians and administrators.

Meanwhile, perhaps the most urgent requirement is to improve the environment in the operating theatre for the patient with a ruptured aneurysm without any loss of efficiency. The dehumanisation of the procedure is not only dreadful for the patient but also bad for the morale and education of the medical and nursing people involved. Probably the best answer would be some form of simple ultrasound screening for aneurysms, followed by elective operations with an expected low mortality and good long-term results.

The Way Ahead

Centralisation of health-care services may well be the best way forward, particularly in a specialist field, such as vascular surgery. Inevitably, many patients will have to travel long distances to get to these highly expensive specialist centres. The health-care economists want to create ever-larger specialist tertiary care hospitals and close small local hospitals. But it is the small local hospitals that patients like, because of the friendliness and ease of visiting for loved ones. This is another dilemma that is difficult to resolve but perhaps it will be possible to arrive at a compromise – with centres of expertise complemented by local hospitals for routine cases.

It is certainly true that there are now some hospitals which are so huge and impersonal that it is impossible for staff to feel any loyalty or sense of belonging. As leaders from Alexander the Great onwards have understood, an army can only be managed efficiently by using a system of small units with identified leaders and hierarchical authority. The same is true of almost any institution. Much of the bureaucracy that goes on in the NHS is a wicked waste of money, paper and time, and could be scrapped without anybody noticing it.

Smaller units in a large institution need to work together in emergencies, such as epidemics or major catastrophes, and this is especially true of intensive and all critical care. Demarcation lines between departments should be ignored in life-and-death situations. Yet, at present, we have a situation where a child can die in an ambulance because there is no paediatric intensive care bed available. This is a scandal – why wasn't an adult intensive care bed used instead? In another outrageous case, an older child was brought to hospital by his father, who believed he had the rapidly fatal disease meningoccocal meningitis. The doctor agreed that this was a likely diagnosis but, instead of giving the simple emergency treatment of penicillin, sent the patient to another hospital with a children's ward. Vital time was thus lost and the boy died. In the old days the ward sister would just have put up another bed and told the doctor to give penicillin. Now we have health and safety rules and fire regulations which might make this difficult. These regulations are used as an excuse to avoid doing what any hospital should have as its first priority – taking care of the sick who come to its doors.

Another problem is that there has been an unexpected increase in hospital emergency admissions. This is largely due to the ever-increasing elderly population and the excessive workload borne by general practitioners. The widespread closure of beds has caused shortages that have crippled every major hospital. More money for patient care will be needed if we are to provide a decent National Health Service. Taxpayers should be asked whether they are prepared to pay more in taxes to improve the NHS. I expect the answer would only be yes if there was also an absolute commitment to reducing to a minimum the present superstructure of managerial staff.

The critical shortage of intensive care beds has recently been highlighted in the press by sad tales of cancelled major operations, turning away of precious donor organs, and the shunting of a dying child across the Pennines. To cancel an operation at the last minute causes anguish for the patient and their whole family, and, if the disease is life-threatening, postponement may result in death. I was once asked what would happen if there were fifty serious casualties from a bomb explosion on a bus outside our hospital. I am sure the staff would be galvanised into action and the 'Dunkirk spirit' would suddenly appear. Extra beds would be put up, nurses with previous experience of critical care would step forward from different parts of the hospital, and word would get round to retired nurses at home in the area. Doctors would all pull together, no matter what their speciality, and I expect even the corps of administrators would drop their clipboards and help with bandages and the fetching of blood. Why can we not respond in a similar manner to small-scale emergencies?

I would suggest that there are three main reasons: lack of critical care beds; the loss of highly trained nurses, due to the stress of continuous working in busy intensive care wards; and the vested interests that want to maintain boundaries around very highly specialised critical care units.

The first problem requires money, but the other two need a change in nurses' training, and – much more difficult – a shift in the attitude of some doctors and nurses. Critical care ranges from the very stressful intensive care of children, neurological cases and general medicine and surgery, to less demanding coronary care, recovery from routine surgery and high dependency. Usually each of these facilities is totally separate.

I believe the solution is to establish a multi-disciplinary training course for nurses covering all aspects of critical care; to rotate nurses between the separate units to widen and maintain their experience and interest and relieve stress; to ensure that when the most appropriate unit is full, the patient is looked after in one of the other units, with staff capable of moving temporarily; and to maintain the high-quality specialist skills that currently exist in each unit with a core of experienced nurses and doctors. These measures would ensure that the doors of major hospitals would remain open; serious operations would not be cancelled at the last moment; desperately needed donor organs would not be turned away; and dying patients would not be sent long distances in search of a special bed.

One of the central questions facing health-care professionals is: who should receive expensive, high-tech medical procedures when resources are limited? The change in society resulting from two parents working and the decline of the extended family has resulted in a disastrous loss of traditional community living. Many parents do not look after their children because of other commitments; likewise children often are unwilling to take care of their parents in later life. The management of increasing numbers of old people is already a major concern in all developed countries: many elderly patients are kept alive in soulless institutions, unable to move independently, with increasing dementia – a sad way to spend their final years.

Children with gross physical and mental defects used to die at birth; now the brilliance of neo-natal intensive care permits many of these babies to survive. Some of them then require full-time care for the rest of their lives – which can be long – and yet they may be incapable of normal human contact and suffer constant pain. Patients demand cosmetic surgery under the NHS and expect high-tech remedies for infertility. Genetic engineering to cure disease or eliminate bad genes is just beginning – rather like flying at the time of the Wright brothers. Soon the Boeing 747 of molecular medicine will be with us, bringing a host of new ethical worries. These developments raise awkward questions which are often deliberately ignored.

In some countries the priorities are simply dictated by the bank balance of the patient (or his insurers). This should not be the case in the National Health Service. Oregon in the United States has grasped this very difficult nettle. The state has a panel of citizens, doctors and government officials who categorise disease according to priority based on expected quality of life. To take two extreme examples, a child with appendicitis would have high priority for admission to a surgical ward and immediate treatment, while an elderly person who has had a stroke and develops kidney failure would have low priority for a kidney transplant or having dialysis treatment. Between such extremes, there are many difficult decisions to be made, and the people of Oregon have decided to review the system at regular intervals. Such an arrangement, of course, really amounts to 'rationing' – a word that causes great dismay among politicians and public alike. But, when there is not enough to go round, rationing is the only fair way of distributing what is available. Sooner or later, a similar approach will have to be adopted by all civilised democracies.

Over the last 100 years, we have come a long way in the development of medicine and surgery, and Britain has been at the forefront of many of the advances – antibiotics, endoscopes, joint replacements, imaging scanners, and preventative medicine (including vaccinations), to name but a few. We have played our part in the pioneering of many areas of surgery, especially cardiac surgery and organ transplantation. Many countries are worse off than us. Those of us who work in the NHS should be proud of our achievements but, unless we can provide for those in need in a better way than at present, we will fail in our medical duty to help the sick and keep the doors of our hospitals always open.

Chapter Fourteen
Crystal Ball Gazing

'Twelve voices were shouting in anger, and they were all alike. No question, now, what had happened to the faces of the pigs. The creatures outside looked from pig to man, and from man to pig, and from pig to man again; but already it was impossible to say which was which.' Animal Farm *by George Orwell.*

In this scene the underprivileged animals shivering in the snow watched the dictator pig Napoleon take his favourite sow to dinner with the farmers and eventually they became confused as to who was a pig and who was a farmer.

As the results of organ transplantation improve, so the demand increases. These procedures will never be cheap and the financial considerations are becoming increasingly prominent in the minds of politicians of all nations, even the wealthiest. Keeping records of outcomes in different disease categories for organ transplants will help us in the difficult and painful task of establishing priorities for treatment (or 'rationing').

It is unlikely that there will be a major increase in organ donation from cadavers. Organs are already removed from elderly donors in whom age may have damaged the organs to be transplanted. More public education and a law of presumed consent may have a positive effect on organ donation. But the congestion on our roads (due to too many cars and new driving rules and restrictions) will, one hopes, reduce the number of youngsters killed in road traffic accidents. More organs will be donated by living related and non-related donors, and continued surveillance will be needed to prevent abuse and commercialisation of live organ donation.

Because of this shortage of organs for transplantation, the possibility of removing organs from animals to transplant into man is very attractive, particularly if organs could be used from agricultural animals, such as pigs or sheep. Unfortunately pigs and sheep are very distant from man in terms of biological relationship. The closest species to humans are the other primates and the closest primate is the chimpanzee. But chimpanzees are an endangered species and there would be little public support for using chimpanzees as donors for humans, particularly since they take a long time to reproduce and grow. Baboons are a more common primate species but they do not grow large enough to have organs that would be suitable for most adults. They may also carry viruses that would be dangerous to man – a subject I discuss in more detail below – and many people feel strongly about the use of any primate species.

Cloning and Transplantation

Objections also exist (although less strident) to the possibility of using organs from pigs or other farm animals. This was previously considered a biological impossibility and there was little debate about it, but we are now at the beginning of an exciting revolution in genetic manipulation. Today it is possible to inject human DNA, which will produce human proteins, into the embryo of a pig and make the pig, at least in one minute part, similar to a human.

It seems unlikely that one or two human genes (out of many hundreds of thousands) would be sufficient to make pig organs acceptable to man, but recent cloning experiments have successfully produced a healthy sheep from the nucleus of an adult sheep's cell.

The task of research in xenografting could be likened to

replacing all the parts of a Rolls-Royce engine with those taken from a Ford. Each individual mechanical item would have roughly the same function for the Rolls-Royce and the Ford but the dimensions, the thread of the screws and the whole balance would be different. It is unlikely at the end of a successful and difficult engineering enterprise that the Rolls would go as well with the Ford components as with its own bespoke engine parts.

Dolly the sheep, who was cloned from an adult sheep's cell removed from the mammary gland of the donor at the Roslin Institute in Edinburgh, was undoubtedly the scientific wonder of 1997. She received great media attention and caused President Clinton to demand an urgent scientific report on cloning. The successful application of cloning confounded the predictions of experts who believed that the nucleus of an adult cell would have differentiated too far to have a chance of reverting to the 'totipotent' state required for an egg to develop. Nevertheless, by depriving the cell of oxygen and rendering it quiescent and probably malnourished, the nuclear transfer to an egg of another sheep whose nucleus had been removed was successful. The egg developed into an intact and apparently normal sheep, which has since become pregnant. Dolly had a little lamb in 1998. Delightful and perfect, as far as one can tell, with feet as white as snow.

It had previously been thought that only embryonal cells could revert to the egg state, and that it would always require fertilisation of an egg from specialised sex gonadal cells (the egg from the female and the sperm from the male) for an adult to produce an egg. However, the Roslin researchers demonstrated that, at least in the sheep, a parthenogenesis (or 'virgin birth') could be stage-managed in the laboratory, with a scientist as the test-tube midwife. Having achieved this, the developmental stage still required a surrogate mother – the cloned embryo needed the environment of a foster mother's uterus for it to develop. An interesting thought emanating from these experiments is that the age of the cloned Dolly at birth was not zero but the age of the cells of the ewe from which the donor cell had been removed.

So, what has all this to do with transplantation? Well, the main thrust of xenograft research has been to insert critically important human proteins into pig embryos, using so-called transgenic injection techniques which are technically difficult and often fail. Also, only a limited amount of DNA can be introduced in this way. With cloning techniques, a whole nucleus could be transformed and then the embryo would be identical to the individual from which the nucleus had been removed (with the exception of the egg DNA present in the mitochondria which comes from the female donor of the egg). Using cloning techniques, it should be possible to introduce larger amounts of human DNA into a pig's ovum than previously, and with greater certainty. The cloned pig would still be a pig with transfected human tissue.

The Potential Problems of Animal-to-Human Grafts

There are no technical difficulties in transplanting a pig's heart into a human; the problems are biological. The technique is straightforward, well within the capability of a competent cardiac surgeon. Of course we all want progress to take place in transplantation but I think it would be a tragedy if further xenografts were done before we know more about the science of rejection of xenografts and the biology of the function of animal organs in another species. Progress is being made, however.

Another major concern that has been very prominent in the media is the potential danger of viruses spreading from animals to humans, particularly in an abnormal environment where the patient's natural immunity is depressed by the drugs necessary to prevent rejection. There has been speculation that the AIDS virus, HIV, originally spread from monkeys to humans; and BSE (mad cow disease) is thought to have been transmitted from sheep to cattle to humans, although the evidence for the last stage has not been particularly convincing.

Retroviruses of the type that cause AIDS are present in all mammals. Often they seem to exist as innocent passengers and may even have become incorporated into the stable DNA of individual cells. It has been shown that pig retroviruses can be grown in human cells but we still do not know whether they could cause a disease in man. Some commentators have expressed their fear that a virus could spread not only to the individual patient but from the patient to the community in general. Although most virologists feel that this disastrous scenario is unlikely, it cannot be completely ruled out.

It is never possible to exclude the danger of something which is unknown. In transplantation many risks have been taken, especially by those patients who submitted themselves to new and dangerous operations in the early days. A careful and well-controlled study of animal-to-human organ grafts, whether it be heart, kidney or tissues (such as islet cells to produce insulin) would seem to be justified, once further work has been done to unravel the background biological uncertainties.

The Ethical Questions

Whenever transplantation is discussed, the question 'is it morally acceptable and ethical?' arises. This is an area to be approached with care and trepidation, but it may be helpful to consider the meaning of the phrase 'morally acceptable and ethical' in a historical context.

A few hundred years ago in Western Europe it was regarded as both 'morally acceptable' and 'ethical' to torture and execute those who did not subscribe to the orthodox religion of the state in which they lived. The citizens did not object; in fact, they enthusiastically supported some of the executions.

Many primitive tribes practised cannibalism, and members of the tribe felt no need to be ashamed of their way of life. In more recent times, there have been many dreadful examples of ethnic cleansing endorsed by a majority of the citizens of the nations perpetrating these crimes.

One is therefore driven to conclude that moral and ethical values are determined by the *mores* of a given society at a given time. For example, in our own society, if a patient with terminal kidney disease were offered the chance of a perfectly matched kidney produced in the laboratory from one of his own blood cells, most people would find this highly acceptable. If one stage in the laboratory process involved the use of a surrogate pregnant animal, many would find this unacceptable. And most people would throw up their hands in horror at the thought of a stage in this laboratory process requiring a surrogate human to provide the environment of her womb to nourish a kidney.

Michael Rees, a surgical research fellow visiting Cambridge from the United States, calls this 'the YUK factor' and I think he has hit the nail squarely on the head. For the moment it seems that we must work within the moral and ethical climate dictated by contemporary society so as not to trigger this 'YUK' response in the majority, bearing in mind that some people will tend to reject *any* new idea. However, provided this idea does not induce a hostile response in most people, and considering that it may help people who are ill, in fear and in pain, then it would seem reasonable to proceed with caution.

Not surprisingly, cloning of human cells has been forbidden in many Western countries, including the United Kingdom. The possibility of cloning a whole human being from an adult cell raises many ethical dilemmas. From the point of view of transplantation, a cloned embryo without a brain, but with other vital organs, would be the perfect donor. But no ethical committee would sanction a surrogate mother for a headless embryo (or 'organ preparation') analogous to the headless frogs which have recently been produced. But what if such an 'organ preparation' could be developed in an artificial womb-like environment in the laboratory?

This holds out the possibility of growing organs with a genetic make-up identical to the donor of the nucleus. Such organs would be accepted as if they came from an identical twin and immunosuppressive treatment would not be necessary. So, will it one day be possible to have a 'bespoke' embryo of exactly the same genetic constitution as the donor of the nucleus who might need an organ transplant? If so, we would be faced with the nightmarish scenario of producing an individual just for the sake of having organs for transplantation. The surrogate mother would effectively be acting as a receptacle for a hybrid organ culture. Such a concept has some similarity to the phenomenon of cuckoos throwing out the legitimate eggs of the hens who care for their chicks. The cuckoo reproduces by using surrogate care from the hen, who has been robbed but does not realise that the eggs are not her own.

This may all sound very far-fetched, and I hope it is. But, as I mentioned elsewhere, we already know of parents who have deliberately conceived an extra child just for the purpose of that child being a bone marrow donor for a sibling who has suffered from leukaemia and needs a bone marrow transplant from a well-matched donor. Would it be morally acceptable if the sick sibling suffered from kidney disease so that the child was brought into the world primarily to give a kidney to the brother or sister? What, then, if a heart or liver were needed? These are terrifying questions. Perhaps the whole procedure could be conducted in some kind of tissue culture in which the embryo was allowed to develop all the organs apart from the brain? Like the headless frog? This might avoid the objection of a sentient creature being produced and nurtured, merely to be an organ donor. In *Brave New World* Aldous Huxley predicted that 'test-tube' babies would be produced in cultures according to the requirements of the ruling class. It is possible that the concept of test-tube organs could one day become a reality.

I have raised these questions, not because I have answers to them, but because I think they are deeply relevant to organ transplantation, the ethics of the medical profession, and the moral culture of our society as a whole. To wait until such developments are a *fait accompli* is far worse than anticipating and debating, potential worries. The Kennedy Committee, established by the British government, has set out clinical and practical guidelines for progress in organ grafting from animals to humans.

Although cloning in humans may be scientifically difficult, if the techniques were available they would certainly be used. For example, bereaved parents might wish to reproduce a child killed in a traffic accident. A clone from one of the dead child's cells would produce an identical twin, even though the individual would be born at a different time and would be nurtured differently. The moral pressure to proceed with cloning of a human being under these circumstances would be difficult to resist. But there would be other, much less deserving cases, such as that of a rich person wishing to reproduce his or her genetic make-up in a child, for reasons of pure vanity. We can only hope that our essential generosity of spirit will overwhelm our baser instincts so that we can 'live and let live' in a brave new world of scientific technology.

At present these musings remain the stuff of fantasy. But, as we have seen many times in the recent past, the development of biotechnology is so rapid and advances often occur in unexpected leaps so that science fiction may very quickly turn into reality.

The Goal of Tolerance

As for transplantation, I would expect the goal of tolerance to be approached if not achieved in the near future. In my own department's research we have tried to mimic the tolerance-producing effect of the liver in pigs without transplanting a liver, using the following method. The recipient pig first received a blood transfusion from the donor. This contained bone marrow-derived cells, including stem cells, and at the time of transplantation one large dose of cyclosporin was given to suppress all the potentially aggressive cells in the recipient. A period of two or three days was deliberately left, to allow an engagement to occur between stem cells in the blood transfusion and those in the recipient. (We do not know the details of such an engagement, or even if it occurs.) After this, only six more doses of cyclosporin were given. Half the pigs survived and were still well more than a year later, with good function in their kidney grafts. Their own kidneys had been removed and they were mis-matched for their donors. If they had not had any treatment, the kidneys would have been rejected between seven and ten days after transplantation. We were pleased with the results of these experiments but they couldn't be applied to humans because the doses of cyclosporin were too high to give to human patients.

Then two years ago, at a meeting in Vienna, a young American surgeon, Stuart Knechtle, described experiments in which he had given monkeys three doses of a powerful monoclonal antibody which targeted the immune cells that cause rejection. However, this antibody was special, in that it was chemically linked to a modified diphtheria toxin so that the target cells were destroyed. These three doses permitted most monkeys to accept kidneys permanently and, after a time, to accept skin grafts from the original donors. It seemed that 'taking out' the immune cells for a short period of time allowed new cells to develop in an environment in which the kidney transplant was already working. The graft thus became accepted as if it was part of the animal's own genetic material.

Herman Waldmann, Geoff Hale and Greg Winter working in Cambridge produced and refined a monoclonal antibody called Campath 1H. This has very similar properties in man to the Immunotox used by Knechtle in monkeys. We have been studying this antibody in patients with kidney grafts and after more than a year of observations, have found that most patients given only two doses of the antibody and then maintained on a half dose cyclosporin have excellent function in their grafted kidneys. A longer follow-up will be necessary but the avoidance of corticosteroids, the low dose of cyclosporin and the absence of side effects have been encouraging. The patients are pleased with the treatment, which seems a step on the road towards tolerance. If the good results are maintained this would markedly reduce the drug costs of organ transplantation and would be especially welcomed in developing countries, where cost can be an overwhelming deterrent. I have called this treatment 'almost tolerance' or the Latin equivalent *prope tolerantia.*

Having spent many years in the search for tolerance, I believe principles have now been established that might be applicable to humans. We need an antibody or a drug that will temporarily wipe out immune activity, either by killing or immobilising all the cells that could react against the grafted kidney. Then, as the immune system recovers, the cells should become tolerant of the kidney. This is not an outlandish or extraordinary hypothesis, since, with bone marrow transplantation, tolerance is already required for the graft to take. In bone marrow transplantation the whole body is subjected to a severe onslaught of x-rays or drugs that destroy the entire immune system and the bone marrow. Then, without any immune defences or blood cell-producing capability of his own, the patient is grafted with bone marrow, usually taken from a well-matched blood relative. Even then, there is a danger that the bone marrow of a relative will react against the host when it is in its new environment, producing a 'Graft versus Host' disease which can be severe and even fatal. A delicate balance is required and we are not always able to control it. However, once a bone marrow transplant has been accepted, it can be followed by a kidney from the same donor without any additional drug treatment.

We hope that, in the near future, we may be able to achieve tolerance using an antibody like Campath 1H that depletes the aggressive cells of the immune system without affecting the bone marrow or the stem cells. A blood transfusion (with stem cells) from the donor might be needed to gain maximum effect. Under these circumstances a patient with a kidney or heart graft might need no further immunosuppression or a very small maintenance dose to guard against chronic rejection or the stirring up of a rejection reaction by a virus infection or allergy. The initial depletion of lymphocytes would set the stage and the minimal immunosuppression would fine-tune control. Patients would no longer require dangerous doses of immunosuppressive drugs after they had got through the initiating treatment. If we are ever to develop transplants from animals to man, some form of tolerance conditioning will be necessary. Establishing and understanding this process in grafts between humans would seem to be a sensible first step.

The general pattern of immunosuppression worldwide, for all organ transplants, is to combine a number of agents in small doses so as to get an added immunosuppressive effect, but without the individual side-effects of the different drugs. Thus, azathioprine, corticosteroids and cyclosporin are commonly used together. Each has different major side-effects. Corticosteroids stunt growth, cause roundness of the face and impair the healing of wounds. Azathioprine can inhibit the bone marrow, causing anaemia and a low white blood cell count. Cyclosporin can cause increase in growth of hair and damage the kidney. However, when these three agents are used together most patients can tolerate them reasonably well. Unfortunately acute rejection crises can still occur and these are usually treated with a short course of high-dose steroids or anti-lymphocyte globulin preparations. This powerful form of immunosuppression may lead to infection, particularly with herpes viruses (resulting in severe cold sores). It may also activate cytomegalic virus infection which can cause a temperature and result in specific damage to a variety of organs. And all immunosuppression predisposes a patient to infection and tumour formation.

Despite these worries, most patients do well with organ grafts and, after a time, can be maintained with relatively low-dose immunosuppression. With few exceptions, however, stopping immunosuppression usually leads to acute rejection and chronic rejection which is difficult to detect and can occur insidiously after years of good function of a graft. Many of us working in transplantation feel that the burden of continuous immunosuppression could potentially be lifted, but more research is needed. We have a number of new immunosuppressive agents, powerful monoclonal anti-lymphocyte antibodies and new drugs. Tacrolimus (FK506) and Cellcept (mycophenolate mofetil) have both recently been registered and it is likely that rapamycin will soon also be registered. However, it is important that the addition of these powerful new immunosuppressants doesn't lead to overkill without any benefit to patients.

In the laboratory there are a number of successful models of tolerance – that is, the induction of a state of non-responsiveness in the recipient towards the graft without continued drug dosage. Manipulating the immune system in this way is probably more difficult in humans than in most animals in whom the experiments are being carried out.

Achieving tolerance probably requires an active relationship between donor and recipient, which I have likened to a football match, and the immunosuppressive drugs are necessary to control the 'hooligans' (that is, the active lymphocytes which are of great value in times of 'war' or when the patient is threatened with an infection, but are harmful to a graft). If donor and recipient can engage with each other, like two football teams, then, when the game is finished, the teams shake hands and the graft is accepted. This window of opportunity for immunological engagement (or WOFIE) may be a requirement before a tolerant state can be produced. And it is likely that excessive immunosuppression (in addition to the well-known dangers of infection and malignancy) might prevent the 'football match' from taking place, meaning that tolerance would never occur.

Hopes for the Future

As this book makes clear, my professional interest has been sharply focused on transplantation for many years. I have seen this form of treatment change from a pipe dream to an established fact and then to a major branch of surgery. Because I have always practised a wide range of general surgery, I have been able to move from kidney to pancreas to liver to intestine, and I have done a great deal of experimental work with heart and lungs. With each shift of interest, I have had to learn more about the organs in question and the diseases that affect them. This I have found extremely stimulating. I also enjoy the technical side of surgery, especially evolving new techniques in organ transplantation.

The biology of transplantation will remain a challenge for many years and this is also a great stimulus to continue with research. I hope that it will be possible to retain these interests as long as my health remains good and my hand–eye co-ordination steady. It is difficult for active surgeons reaching retirement age to carry the full burden of a consultant surgeon one day and be condemned to doing nothing the next. It would be more sensible to make some use of our experience for a few years after we reach retirement age. At the end of a career in surgery one has inevitably made many mistakes, and it would certainly benefit patients if this experience could help our successors. Young surgeons in training can always learn from older surgeons in order to avoid repeating the same mistakes, although they will undoubtedly make their own.

Extreme specialisation and new technologies (particularly minimally invasive techniques) are changing the practice of surgery very rapidly. And, as I have indicated, there is a danger that much of surgery will become a form of technology, divorced from the vocational side of medicine that traditionally requires a broad and lengthy medical training.

Over the years, I have trained many young surgeons in general surgery and transplantation. Most have been successful in setting up their own units. Many surgical Fellows from all over the world have visited our department in Cambridge to do research and learn the techniques of organ transplantation. Some have visited for a few days, others for years (the longest for nine years). Sadly, when they return to their own countries they frequently have great difficulty in establishing effective transplantation programmes. This can sometimes be due to local laws or superstitions but it is often because of opposition from colleagues who are jealous because they will be blazing a new surgical trail and the work will inevitably raise their profile. In a profession that is supposed to be devoted to helping suffering humanity, it is surprising how often ambition and personal jealousy can impede the care of the sick. In this respect our profession is, I suppose, no different from any other. But I would like to be able to help some of my ex-Fellows develop their programmes, as a senior colleague who would not be a threat to their own career aspirations.

My ex-surgical Fellows' difficulties also frequently arise because of lack of funds and insufficient understanding of the expensive infrastructure needed to support organ transplantation. The time spent in the operating theatre is only a part, although an extremely important one, of the ongoing process of achieving a life-saving transplant that will provide full rehabilitation for the patient. The care received before and after the procedure is also vital.

From my wife's point of view, it is a very hard life to be married to a surgeon, particularly if he is involved with transplantation. Social functions are often ruined and calls to the operating theatre frequently interrupt the most carefully laid plans. We once had a party in our house for sixty guests whom Patsy had to receive and entertain alone, although she knew only four or five of them.

There have been many failures and disappointments, particularly in the early days of transplantation. At these times my wife's support stopped me despairing and giving the whole thing up (an option which would have been considered sensible by many of my colleagues).

I have had numerous intermittent disputes with bureaucrats in the university, my hospital, and the Department of Health. Incidentally, I had assumed the Department of Health were reasonably familiar with my activities so it was a surprise to receive a congratulatory telegram in June 1986, on the occasion of my knighthood, which referred to my 'services to Obstetrics and Gynaecology'!

In October 1998 I retired from my University Chair. I hope I will be able to carry on participating in the research that has fascinated me for the past forty years and continue my involvement in the care of patients requiring organ transplants. They are very courageous people, and work must continue in order to make their treatment safer and their return to health quicker and more complete.

When I consider the many extraordinary patients I have encountered in my career as a surgeon, I am reminded of Prince Hamlet's words in Act II, Scene 21, of Shakespeare's great play:

> What a piece of work is man
> How noble in reason!
> How infinite in faculty!
> In form and moving how express and admirable!
> In action how like an angel!
> In apprehension how like a God!
> The beauty of the world!
> The paragon of animals . . .

Appendix I
The Main Transplant Organs

The Heart

Although it may appear the simplest of organs the heart is a remarkable pump working continuously from before we are born to the moment of death. It responds to increasing demands and can produce spectacular performance in output of blood in athletes at maximum exertion. There are two separate halves of the heart and four chambers, with a complicated system of valves to ensure that the blood flows in the right direction. From the veins draining the main part of the body, blood goes to the right side of the heart, and is pumped into the lungs to receive fresh oxygen and get rid of carbon dioxide. It is then returned from the lungs to the left side of the heart and from there, under high pressure, the blood is ejected into the main artery of the body, the aorta, to supply first the heart itself (through the coronary arteries) and then the rest of the body – head, arms, trunk and legs.

The heart responds to emotion and has always held a special place in human mythology and culture.

The Lungs

The lungs are two air-filled organs that fill a large part of the chest (the rest of the chest accommodates the heart). The lungs have a dual function: to replenish the blood with oxygen used up in the metabolic activity of the body; and to remove poisonous carbon dioxide that has accumulated as a result of this metabolism. To achieve this exchange of gases, the lungs have an enormous surface area and a powerful mechanism for taking in and expelling gas through the windpipe (or trachea) and its tree-like branches, to the air sacs throughout the lung tissue. This bellows-like activity requires powerful muscles, namely those of the diaphragm. The diaphragm separates the chest from the abdomen and descends towards the abdomen when we breathe in; at the same time the ribs expand so that the chest cavity is enlarged, both in its circumference and in its lower limit. This greatly increases its volume and sucks air into the lungs.

The lungs have a huge circulation of blood. In fact, half the body's total blood volume is pumped by the heart through the lungs and the other half is pumped through the rest of the body. If the air passages are blocked the air sacs collapse and there is a danger of infection leading to pneumonia. Damage to the diaphragm or to the nerves that supply the rib muscles will prevent expansion of the lungs, and a penetrating injury of the chest will cause collapse of the lungs, possibly resulting in a dangerous build-up of pressure which obstructs the action of the heart. The lungs are vital organs, although it is possible to live in reasonable comfort and health with one functioning lung. Any disease that interferes with the mobility of a patient increases susceptibility to infection of the lungs; this is aggravated by anaesthetics and other sedative drugs and the immunosuppressive agents that we give to prevent organ graft rejection. It is therefore not surprising that many disasters in transplantation have ended in death from lung infection.

The Pancreas

This organ, shaped like a large tadpole, has a duct that drains into the duodenum, a part of the intestine close to the stomach.

Through this duct we secrete the important fermenting enzymes that digest fat, proteins and carbohydrates. In addition, scattered throughout the pancreas are clusters of cells called islets, described by Langerhans when he was a young German medical student 100 years ago. The most important cells in the islets are the beta cells which produce insulin.

Why the islets are embedded in the pancreas in all mammals is not understood. In some fishes they are separated from the pancreas, but in mammals there appears to be a close interrelationship between the minute blood vessels of the islets and those of the rest of the pancreas which produce the digestive juices. Insulin is normally secreted into these blood vessels and passes first to the liver (where the insulin controls the glucose level in the blood and the laying down of the carbohydrate glycogen, which is used as an energy store).

Failure to secret insulin results in diabetes, a disease which causes patients to become emaciated, with an enormous hunger and thirst. They lose weight and drink large quantities of fluid, to compensate for the fluid loss from the kidneys due to sugar secretion which takes fluid with it into the urine. The secondary effects of diabetes are not fully understood but they can cause a great deal of damage to the eyes, kidneys and bladder, as well as abscesses and gangrene of the extremities. These changes have not been shown to be reversed by a successful vascularised pancreatic graft, although the condition does not get any worse. By the time a diabetic receives a pancreas graft, they usually also require a kidney graft and the disease is so advanced that the patient's quality of life may not be greatly improved. Nevertheless there have been some remarkable exceptions, especially in young patients.

There has been intensive work for the last thirty years to try to treat diabetes by transplanting the islets alone, without the rest of the pancreas. This has the obvious attraction of avoiding a major operation, since the islets can be injected from a syringe. Although this seems to be a satisfactory technique in rat and mouse experiments it has been very disappointing when tried in humans and has not resulted in any long-term successes.

The results of pancreas transplantation for diabetes are steadily improving. Most of the patients selected for pancreas transplantation were in the final stages of prolonged suffering from diabetes – often with impairment of vision or even blindness and damage to nerves and arteries. When these patients developed diabetic kidney failure and required a kidney transplant, there was a strong argument for also grafting the pancreas from the same donor, since the patient would require long-term immunosuppression and the pancreas would presumably prevent the diabetic kidney disease from affecting the renal graft. In some patients these positive expectations were fulfilled but the pancreas is not a surgically friendly organ. Besides producing insulin, the pancreas also provides the ferments or enzymes that dissolve proteins, fats and carbohydrates. If this ferment containing pancreatic juice leaks outside the intestinal tract, it causes severe damage to whatever tissue with which it comes in contact. Patients on immunosuppression tend to heal their wounds badly and are susceptible to infection, so leakage of pancreatic juice is a common complication after pancreas transplantation.

Attempts have been made to stop the secretion of pancreatic juice by injecting a rubber glue into the pancreatic duct, or the pancreatic juice can be drained into a loop of bowel or the bladder. This latter route was preferred by many centres, despite theoretical objections that it might cause inflammation of the bladder. Currently pancreatic transplantation together with kidney transplantation is popular in North America but less so in Europe due to the complications mentioned; nevertheless, results are improving and new immunosuppressive drugs seem to be contributing to the better outcome of patients.

The Liver

The liver is a large organ occupying a central position in the body. It can be regarded as a major chemical plant, producing most of the vital proteins and other substances that we need to stay healthy. It also removes toxins from the blood, and detoxifies many drugs that would otherwise cause general damage. The liver produces bile which is a fluid for the excretion of bile pigment (a waste product from broken-down red blood cells). However, bile also contains bile salts which are essential for the absorption of fat in the food we eat. In addition, the liver contains numerous scavenger cells which engulf and destroy bacteria that may leak into the bloodstream, especially from the bowel.

When the liver fails, all these vital functions are disrupted. If the main bile duct or small bile ducts in the liver are obstructed the patient becomes jaundiced and the bile salts accumulating in the blood cause itching which can be intolerable. The inability to absorb fat leads to malnutrition, and lack of bile in the intestine leads to a poor appetite. Drugs in normal doses can become highly toxic; a small glass of wine can cause a patient with severe liver disease to become semi-conscious.

Cirrhosis hardens the liver and blocks the blood going into the liver from the intestine. This leads to veins in the stomach and gullet becoming engorged. Together with the increased tendency to bleed (because clotting factors are not being produced by the damaged liver), this can result in catastrophic haemorrhage from the gullet which is a common cause of death in liver failure. The inability to produce albumen (one of the main proteins in the blood) results in fluid accumulating in the legs and abdominal cavity. This is aggravated by high pressure in the veins of the abdomen. It is almost miraculous to see how all these symptoms of severe liver disease are rapidly reversed by a well-functioning transplanted liver.

In the ancient Babylonian and Etruscan civilisations the liver played a central role in religion. The Etruscans had a special priest, called the 'harospex', who inspected the livers of sacrificed animals. From their appearance, he foretold the outcome of battles and determined good and bad omens concerning all aspects of life.

The Kidneys

A pair of organs, one in each loin, the kidneys are extremely efficient filters of the blood, removing waste products and concentrating them and also producing a hormone called erythropoietin which is vital for the production of red blood cells. Each kidney contains about a million tiny organ systems called nephrons (each nephron consisting of a filtering glomerulus and a tubule). The tubules selectively re-absorb important constituents from the blood, leaving only excretory products and excess water to be voided in the urine. Each kidney has a large artery and an even larger vein and the urine is drained via the kidney into the ureter and then to the bladder. When the kidneys fail, fluid accumulates in the body, red cells are not produced (so there is marked anaemia), and the patient's blood pressure usually rises (because the damaged kidneys release peptides that cause arterial spasm and high blood pressure).

Most of these symptoms can be overcome by washing the blood through an artificial kidney dialysing machine, or by peritoneal dialysis (in which fluid is introduced into the abdominal cavity through a tube). After the waste products have left the blood and the constituents the patient needs have entered the blood, the fluid containing excretory matter is drained out through the same tube. Recurrent haemodialysis requires needles to be placed in special veins that have been joined to arteries (usually in the arm), and peritoneal dialysis requires an in-dwelling tube in the abdominal cavity. Both these sites can develop complications – especially infection and thrombosis of the blood vessels and blockage of the peritoneal dialysing tube.

A patient with a normally functioning kidney graft has a much better quality of life than can be achieved by dialysis. In addition, he or she does not require supplements of erythropoietin to maintain a normal red blood cell count. When a kidney is transplanted it is usually placed in the pelvis, which is easier for surgical access than the normal position in the loin. The pelvic bones give some protection, though not as much as that provided by the fat, ribs and muscles that surround the kidney in the normal position. A patient with a kidney transplant therefore has to be careful to avoid blows to the lower abdomen and sports that involve bodily contact.

The Bowel

Obtaining nourishment from food, and disposing of the indigestible residue, are the tasks of the gastrointestinal tract. Once we have swallowed our food, we tend to think of it being churned in the stomach, rather like clothes in a washing machine, as the process of digestion begins. This involves breaking down the food into its smaller constituents, like glucose and amino acids and small particles of fat which can be absorbed into the blood and then further processed by the liver.

Most of the digestive process occurs in the long coiled tube called the small bowel. The first part of the small bowel is the duodenum. This receives bile and juice from the pancreas which are important in digestion. Loss of the small bowel used to result in death but it is now possible for some patients to be fed through a vein by a process rather akin to dialysis for kidney disease. This intravenous feeding requires obsessive care on the part of the patient, the doctors and nurses to ensure that the tube in the vein does not get blocked or infected. It also severely impairs the patient's quality of life because the feeding is very slow and time-consuming. This is why transplantation of the small bowel is such an appealing option.

However, the bowel is unfortunately very susceptible to rejection (rather like skin). A small amount of damage, that could be repaired in the kidney or liver, may breach the surface lining of the bowel and allow bacteria to enter the patient's bloodstream, with disastrous results (especially as the patient's ability to combat infection will be depressed by immunosuppressive drugs).

The surgery involved in transplanting the bowel is not particularly difficult. The artery and vein separating the graft must be joined to appropriate vessels in the recipient and the ends of the bowel joined to the stomach and colon, if the patient has a colon, or brought out as an ileostomy stoma (an external opening in the patient's abdomen) if the colon has also been removed.

The colon leading to the rectum and anus is the last portion of the gastrointestinal tract. Food has already been absorbed but the colon absorbs excess water and acts as a reservoir for the stools. This is a very useful function but not vital. Thus, patients can survive in remarkably good health with the whole of the colon removed and a permanent stoma. Colon transplantation has not so far been practised because of the dangers of immunosuppression.

Appendix II
Glossary

Antibody Protein produced in the body in response to an antigen. Protects from infection and can destroy grafts

Antigen Substance that stimulates an antibody, e.g. red blood group proteins A and B, tissue type substances, viruses and bacteria

Graft or transplant Tissue or organ moved from its original position to survive and function elsewhere

Autograft Graft from one part of the body to another part of the same body

Allograft Graft from one individual to another of the same species

Isograft Graft from one identical twin to another or from one member of an inbred animal strain to another of the same strain

Xenograft Graft from one species to another

Stem cells Cells in the bone marrow and blood which give rise to red blood cells, white blood cells and platelets

Bone marrow Tissue in centre of bones which manufactures both red and white blood cells and blood platelets that are needed for the blood to clot

Lymphocytes White blood cells especially involved in graft rejection. They act by producing antibodies (B lymphocytes) and killing directly (T lymphocytes)

Tissue types Concerned with graft rejection. Typing involves identification of the human lymphocyte antigens (HLA). These are numerous and therefore between unrelated individuals a perfect match is unlikely (e.g. 1 in 2,000). There will be a half match between parent and child. With siblings 1 in 4 are perfectly matched, 1 in 4 have no match and 2 in 4 are half-matched

Immunity The body's defence against infection and grafts. Once experienced, a second encounter with the same bacteria or a graft from the same individual is destroyed very quickly

Immunosuppression Depression of the immune system by drugs or antibodies

Anti-lymphocyte antibodies Produced by injection of, for example, human lymphocytes into a rabbit and using the rabbit's serum (ALS) for immunosuppressive treatment. Monoclonal anti-lymphocyte antibodies are refined antibodies, the result of genetic engineering, which act against a single molecule target (as opposed to ALS which act against many targets)

Tolerance Natural or artificial manipulation of the immune system so that the individual accepts grafts that would otherwise be rejected

Appendix III

Key Dates in the History of Transplantation

1944 Thomas Gibson and Peter Medawar demonstrated rejection as an immunological process

1953 David Hume performed a series of kidney transplants in humans

1954 First identical twin transplants carried out by Joseph Murray at the Peter Bent Brigham Hospital in Boston

1956 Demonstration of Medawar's tolerance findings

1959 Paper in *Nature* by Schwartz and Damashek on inhibition of antibody production in rabbits treated with 6MP

1960 First use of 6MP at the Royal Free Hospital, London, in patients with kidney transplants

1962 First use of azathioprine in clinic at the Peter Bent Brigham Hospital in Boston

1963 First liver transplant in the world performed by Thomas Starzl in Denver

1964 Transplant of kidney from chimpanzee to man by Keith Reemtsma in New Orleans
Transplant of chimpanzee heart to man by James Hardy at Mississippi Medical Center

1967 First heart transplant performed by Christiaan Barnard in South Africa

1977 First use of cyclosporin in Cambridge

1985 Baby Fae received a baboon heart transplant in the United States
Ben Hardwick had his first liver transplant in Cambridge

1986 First combined heart, lung and liver transplant carried out in collaboration with Papworth surgeons

1993 First successful six-organ graft in Cambridge : liver, pancreas, kidney, stomach, duodenum and small bowel; patient well five years later

Index

Addenbrooke's Hospital 66, 73-5, 78–9, 92, 96–8, 100–1, 107, 115–16, 130, 159, 163, 169, 172, 189
Alexander, Graeme 157
Alexandre, Guy 64
Alistair 76–8
allografts 22–3, 30, 32, 41, 102, 199
anaesthetics 9, 40, 61, 83, 111, 131, 152, 163, 167, 170–1, 192
anatomy, study of 16–18, 28–9, 147, 166
Andropov, Y.V. 141
aneurysms 168–72
Animal Farm 110, 177
animals
  regulations governing experiments on 60
  transmission of disease from 180–1
  use of organs from *see* xenografting
  see also baboons; cattle; chimpanzees; dogs; mice; pigs; rabbits; rats
Ashbourne, John 132
autografts 22–3, 30, 40, 199
azathioprine 49, 52–4, 56, 89, 115, 129, 186, 201

baboons, use of 59, 151, 178, 202
Baird, Betty 122, 127
Barnard, Christiaan 81, 128–9, 202
Bearstead, Jane 117–18
Bell, Peter 90–1
Bellany, John 149
Billingham, Rupert 23, 25, 84
Billroth, Theodor 97
Binns, Richard 84
blood clotting factors 103–4, 195

blood loss 77–80, 99–100, 134, 168
blood supplies 103–4
bone marrow transplantation 41, 82, 183, 185–6, 200
Borel, Jean 115
bowel transplantation 130, 132–3, 154, 197–8
Bradfield, John 136
brain (or brain-stem) death 58, 61, 65–8, 124–5
Brendl, Walter 81
Brent, Leslie 23, 25, 42, 84
Brian 151–2
Bridewell, Gordon 102–3
Bright's disease 1, 32, 43, 75
Brock, Russell 7–10, 91, 155
BSE 180
Buckston Browne Farm 38–9, 41, 55
bureaucracy 111, 136, 164, 173–4, 190
Burroughs Wellcome Laboratories 48
BW57-322 49; *see also* azathioprine

Cambridge and Cambridge University 92, 73–4, 135–7, 189
Campath 1H 185–6
Calne, Patsy (author's wife) 14–18, 37, 39–40, 48–9, 51, 53, 91, 105, 123, 141–2, 189–90
Carrel, Alexis 30
cattle, use of 23–5, 34, 41; *see also* BSE
Chan, Celia 110, 131
children
  author's 19, 39, 48, 51, 53, 91–2, 139
  author's paintings of 149–51
chimpanzees, use of 59, 178, 202
China 58, 109–13, 144–5
cirrhosis 102, 109, 127, 157, 159, 195
Clarke, William 169–72
Clinton, President 179
cloning 178–80, 182–3
Clot, J.-P. 84
college system at Cambridge 136–9
complaints about health care 162–3
consent to operations 33, 43, 58, 61–4, 125–6, 133
  presumed 62–3, 177
corticosteroids 91, 122, 185–6
Crick, Francis 27
criminals, organs taken from 52, 58, 65, 71, 112, 142
Crock, Harry 29
cyclosporin 109, 115–21, 129, 154, 184–7, 202

Damashek, William 41, 201
Dausset, Jean 46
Davies, Hugh 84
Davies, Laura 130–2

death, definition of and criteria for 58, 64–8, 98, 125
Delve, Brad 153–4
Dempster, William 30, 38, 41–2
diabetes 117–18, 120, 161, 166, 193–4
dialysis 31, 43–4, 53, 74, 117, 159, 196
DNA 27, 48, 178, 180
dogs, use of 30, 38, 40–2, 49–50, 53, 84–5, 93, 95, 116
Dolly the sheep 178–9
donor organs 30, 34, 43, 52, 152, 177–8
  journeys to collect 105–8
  removal of 56–63, 68–72, 99–100
  see also living donors
Duffet, Roger 141

Mr Eckhoff 8–9
ecological balance 144–5
Elion, Trudy 48–9
Ellis, Harold 19, 56, 73
ethical issues 33, 58, 60–2, 68–9, 134, 136, 176, 181–3
Evans, David 74

Faulwasser, Sister 8
Fisons Pharmaceuticals 121
FK506 118–21, 151, 154, 187
Franklin, Rosalin 27
French contributions to transplantation 46–7, 58
Friend, Peter 131
Fujisawa (company) 118–19, 121, 151
fund-holding GPs 164
funding for research 136

gangrene 152, 193
Gardner's syndrome 131, 153
Garnier, Henri 84
general practice 164, 167
Ghurkas, the 12–15
Gibson, Thomas 22–4, 201
Gillespie, Fulton (Jock) 123
globulin 41, 102, 187
glomerolonephritis 43, 117; *see also* Bright's disease
Goodwin, William 54
Gordon Hospital 59, 73
Gorer, Peter 42
Gowans, James 85, 87
Graham-Jones, Oliver 59–60
Guasp, Paco Torrent 28–9
Guy's Hospital and Medical School 1–2, 5–6, 8, 160–1

Hale, Geoff 185
Hall, Jenny 150
Hallett Prize 18
Hamburger, Jean 40, 46–7
Hardwick, Andrew 127
Hardwick, Ben 124–7, 202
Hardy, James 202
Harkness Foundation fellowship 48, 51
Harvard Medical School 30–1, 40, 48, 51
Hašek, Milan 25
heart, the 66–7, 191

heart/lung machines 66, 128, 162, 166
heart transplantation 50, 81, 127–9
hepatitis 39, 102–4, 158–9
Herrick, Richard and Ronald 32
heterotopic operations 93, 95
Hitchings, George 48–9
Hong Kong 12–14, 110–13
Hopewell, John 38–9, 42–3
Horrobin, David 26
Hoyer, Jochem 68–9
Hufnagel, Charlie 31–2
Hume, David 31–2, 42, 51–2, 57–8, 201
Hyatt, Stephen 131–2

identical twins and triplets 23–4, 32–4, 54, 68, 132–3, 183, 201
immune systems 23–5, 40, 185–7
immunosuppression 33–4, 45–6, 51, 53–6, 58, 76, 94, 97, 109, 115–22, 126–7, 129, 133, 182, 186–8, 192, 200
  natural 122
Imuran 49; *see also* azathioprine
India 69, 143
insulin 60, 117, 181, 193–4
intensive care facilities 150–1, 163, 173–5
International Transplantation Society 58, 101, 119
Irvine, Bill 55
Irvine, Sir Miles 133
Iwatsuki, Shun 90

Jamieson, Neville 131
Japan 13–14, 66, 118–19
jaundice 39, 94, 101, 124, 126, 153, 195
Jehovah's Witnesses 104
Jonathan 1–2, 43
Jones, Philip and Peter 132–3
Joysey, Valerie 75

Kamada, Naoshi 84
Kennedy Committee 183
Keynes, Richard 83
kidney disease 1–2, 31, 43–4, 116–17
  in donors 33, 44
kidney transplantation 2, 30–3, 38, 40–7, 49–50, 52–9, 74–5, 80, 89, 108–9, 116, 127, 129, 139, 185, 193–4, 196, 201
King's College Hospital 97–8, 100, 102, 125
Dr Kitikara 141
Knechtle, Stuart 184–5
Kohler, Thomas 33
Kolff, William 31
Kostakis, Alkis 115–16
Kuss, René 46–7, 58
Kwok, David 110

Large, Paul 6
Le Gros Clarke, Sir Wilfred and Lady 18, 22, 37

legal issues 33, 62–70 *passim*, 124, 165
Lindop, Mike 110, 112
listening to patients 10
Lister, Joseph 28
liver transplantation 50, 83–4, 88–9, 91, 93–105, 111–12, 120, 122, 125, 127, 134, 149–52, 157, 159, 184, 195, 201–2
  combined with other grafts 127, 130
  logistics of 99–100, 108–9
  procedure for 98–100
liver transplantation units 108
liver trauma 77–9, 100
living donors 52, 56, 68–9, 72; *see also* relatives
London Zoo 59–60
Loughridge, Lavinia 56
Lower, Richard 53, 129
Lu, Earl 149
lung transplantation 50, 127–9
lymphocytes 33–4, 40, 119–21, 186, 200
  anti-lymphocyte preparations 81, 151, 187, 200
Lysenko, Trofim 25, 85

McGewan, Molly 75
McLeod, Nigel 75–6
Marcos, Ferdinand and Imelda 140–1
Margreiter, Raimond 82–3
Medawar, Jean 22
Medawar, Peter 2, 21–5, 33–4, 42, 47, 75, 81, 84–7, 201
media, the 123–8, 130, 134
Medical College of Virginia 51–2
Merrill, John 31–2
mice, use of 24–5
Milne, Malcolm 56
Milstein, Ben 8, 76
Milstein, Caesar 33
Mitchison, Avrin 42
monkeys, use of 129, 180, 185
Moore, Francis 31–2, 47, 50–1, 53–4, 84, 93, 95–7
Morris, Peter 139
multiple transplantation 127–32, 202
Murray, Joseph 32–3, 41, 47–51, 53–4, 89, 201

National Health Service 11–16, 159–65, 173–6
Necker Hospital (Paris) 46
negligence, medical 165, 167
Neil, John 75
Nobel Prizes 33, 48, 54
Northwick Park Hospital 74–5
Nuffield Orthopaedic Centre 18, 160
nurses 150–1, 160–3, 174–5

Ochiai, Takenori 118–19
Ona, Ike 139–40
originality in science 25–6
orthotopic operations 53, 84, 93, 95, 116
O'Shea, Eileen 152–3
Owen, Ray 24

Oxford and Oxford University 17, 21–2, 138

painting, author's 149–55
pancreas, the 117, 157, 192–4
Panorama 67, 125
Papworth Hospital 127–9, 202
Pausawasdi, Arun 142–3
payment for organs or organ removal 64, 69, 178
Peacock, Joe 84
Peart, Stanley 55–6
Peter Bent Brigham Hospital 30–3, 40–1, 47–54 *passim*, 57, 84, 201
Petrovski, Professor 86–7
Philippines Kidney Society 139–40
Pichlmayr, Professor 152
pigs, use of 34, 84, 88, 93, 95, 116, 122, 178, 180, 184
population explosion 143–5
Porter, Ken 41, 55–6, 89–90
private practice 137, 164

quality of life, patients' 71–2, 117, 153, 176, 193, 197
Quist, George 40

rabbits, use of 22–3, 34, 41
Radcliffe Infirmary 17
Rainey, Tamara 150
Ranson, Ron 149
Rantzen, Esther 126–7
rapamycin 121, 187
rationing 172, 175–7
rats, use of 38, 84, 115–16, 118–19, 121–2
re-transplant operations 126, 130, 134
Reemtsma, Keith 59, 202
Rees, Michael 182
Reitz, Bruce 129
rejection 23, 32–4, 41–2, 50, 54, 84, 94, 115, 119, 126, 129, 133, 151–4, 157, 180, 184, 186–7, 197
relatives, grafting between 68–70, 108–9, 159, 183, 186
religion 27–8, 88
resuscitation 61, 63–4
Richmond (Virginia) 51–2, 129
Dr Ringe 134
Romesa 150
Roser, Bruce 84
Roslin Institute 179
Royal Army Medical Corps 11–14
Royal College of Surgeons 38, 143
  fellowship of 16–18, 37
  of Thailand 141–2
Royal Free Hospital 37, 39, 42–3, 45, 55, 92, 201
Royal Marsden Hospital 40
Royal Society 85, 144
Russell Flint, Francis and William 148–9
Russian science 85–7

St Mary's Hospital (London) 55–6

St Vincent Hospital (Melbourne) 73–4
St Vincent's Hospital (New York) 158
Samson, Derek 102
Sandoz (company) 115–17
Schwartz, Robert 41, 201
Scott, Brian 158–9
Scribner, Belding 53
Sehgal, Suren 121
Semmelweis, Ignaz 28
Shaldon, Stanley 43
sheep, cloning of 178–9
Sherlock, Sheila 37, 39
Shumway, Norman 52–3, 129
shunts (between artery and vein) 53
Simonsen, Morton 30, 38
Singapore 11–12, 15–16, 18
6MP (6-Mercaptopurine) 31, 41–2, 45–6, 48–9, 53, 115, 201
six-organ transplant 131–2, 202
skin grafting 22–5, 32, 41, 117, 185
Slapak, Maurice (Taffy) 72
Sloan-Kettering Institute 102
Slome, David 38, 40
Smith, Michael 110, 112
Smith, Winnie 101
Smithers, David 40
specialisation in health care 165–8, 173–4, 189
Stanford University 52–3, 129
Starzl, Thomas 42, 54, 59, 88–91, 93–6, 118–19, 122, 126, 130, 201
Steadman, Evan 157–8
steroids 54, 89, 129, 151, 187
Summerlin, W.T. 102
surrogate mothers 182–3
Szuber, Chester and Patti 70

Tacrolimus 187; *see also* FK506
television 124–6, 130; *see also* media
Terasaki, Paul 109
Terblanche, John 84
test-tube babies 183
Thailand 141–3
That's Life 126
Thomas, Donald 54
Thompson, Davina 127–8
Thorn, George 31–2
tissue typing 75, 109, 200
tolerance 84, 122, 184–8, 200
training, medical 165–7, 175, 188–9
Transplant Games and Transplant Olympics 72
transplantation
  author's interest in 1–2, 22, 38, 188
  early experiments in 24, 30–5
  see also under individual organs
trauma, response to 31; *see also* liver trauma
Trinity College 136–8
Trinity Hall 137–9
Dr Tsakis 131
tuberculosis 13, 143, 160
twins 24, 34, 40; *see also* identical twins

ultrasound scanning 169, 172
United States, author's visits to 47–53, 59
University College (London) 42

valve operations 7, 31
vascular surgery 32
ventilation 63–7, 98, 157
Veterans' Administration Hospital (Denver) 89
viruses and virus infection 180–1, 187

Waddel, Bill 89
waiting lists 164
Waldmann, Herman 185
Wallace, Alfred 86
Wallwork, John 128
waste in the NHS 163–5
Watanapa, Dr Prasit 142
Watson, Frank 39, 41
Watson, James 27
Waxman, Byron 33
Westminster Hospital 56–7, 59
White, David 115–16
Wildsmith, Alan and Monica 159
Williams, Roger 97–8, 108, 127
Wilson's Disease 151
Wingfield Morris Hospital 18–19
Winter, Greg 185
WOFIE 188
Woodruff, Michael 33–5, 42
Woodward, Shaun 126–7
Wyeth (company) 121

x-ray crystallography 27
x-rays, treatment with 40–1, 56, 186
xenografting 30, 35, 52, 151, 178–81, 186

'yuk factor' 182

Zimmermann, Franz 84
Zukoski, Charlie 42, 31